CARDIOLOGY RESEARCH AND CLINICAL DEVELOPMENTS

A CLOSER LOOK AT CARDIOVASCULAR DISEASES AND RISK FACTORS

CARDIOLOGY RESEARCH AND CLINICAL DEVELOPMENTS

Additional books in this series can be found on Nova's website under the Series tab.

Additional e-books in this series can be found on Nova's website under the eBooks tab.

CARDIOLOGY RESEARCH AND CLINICAL DEVELOPMENTS

A CLOSER LOOK AT CARDIOVASCULAR DISEASES AND RISK FACTORS

FARIS VAN KILSDONK
EDITOR

nova
Medicine & Health
New York

Library of Congress Cataloging-in-Publication Data

ISBN: 978-1-53613-939-6

Published by Nova Science Publishers, Inc. † New York

CONTENTS

PREFACE

In recent decades, obesity levels have increased worldwide, thus also increasing the prevalence of morbid obesity. This type of obesity is associated with a large number of comorbidities that increase the mortality risk of the patients who suffer it. In this compilation, the authors examine treatment options for this type of population. Bariatric surgery has proven to be an effective method, generating large weight reductions and improving cardiovascular risk factors, thus increasing the life expectancy of patients who undergo it. However, this surgery also has certain disadvantages. In recent years, several studies have also determined that performing exercise at high intensities and adding resistance training to an exercise program generates greater losses of fat mass and reductions in cardiovascular risk factors compared to traditional recommendations. Additionally, endothelial dysfunction is a well-described precursor to the development of clinically overt coronary and peripheral artery disease, and is present early in the course of the disease. It reflects not only the global atherosclerotic status, but also the degree of rigidity of the whole artery system. The measurement of endothelial function could therefore represent an additional prognostic marker of cardiovascular risk. The authors stress the necessity to find methods that could evaluate the endothelial function in an easier and less invasive way. Following this, the authors review the relationship between cardiovascular risk factors, systemic circulatory diseases and inner ear disorders, particularly focusing on the involvement of cardiovascular factors in the pathogenesis of sudden sensorineural hearing. The inner ear may be impaired by vascular affections since it is supplied by a terminal blood flow and has a sustained metabolic activity. It has been reported that the function of labyrinthine vessels can be influenced by several local factors such as perivascular sympathetic innervation, arterial systemic blood pressure and labyrinth liquids pressure ratio, antidiuretic hormone receptors, endothelial dysfunction and ionic transport mechanisms. Next, the current evidence of obesity-related comorbidities is reviewed, along with the cardiovascular risk factor index after different bariatric approaches. Bariatric surgery has been shown to be effective in achieving and maintaining weight change and reducing obesity-related comorbidities. Malabsorptive procedures have been associated with the greatest reduction of cardiovascular risk and the greatest improvement in obesity-related comorbidities. On the other hand, the lowest improvement is seen after restrictive procedures. In conclusion, cardiovascular diseases are the leading cause of death in both men and women. There has been steady decline in mortality from cardiovascular diseases in middle-aged men based on recent data from the National Health and Nutrition Examination Surveys, but for women this rate has remained relatively unchanged. Although there are similarities in most classic risk factors in men and women, the varying implications of these risk factors for both genders are examined.

Chapter 1 - In recent decades, obesity levels have increased worldwide, increasing the prevalence of morbid obesity. This type of obesity is associated with a large number of comorbidities that increase the mortality risk of the patients who suffer it. Therefore, it is necessary to apply a treatment to this type of population. Bariatric surgery has proven to be an effective method, generating large weight reductions and improving cardiovascular risk factors, thus increasing the life expectancy of patients who undergo it. However, this surgery has certain disadvantages. On the one hand, some factors, such as total weight, comorbidities associated with obesity or low cardiorespiratory fitness, are associated with a greater number of surgical complications and a higher rate of intra and postoperative mortality. On the other hand, one of the most common problems after surgery is the weight regain, which is associated with a relapse in different comorbidities, such as diabetes mellitus.

Physical activity has been proved to be an effective tool for reducing total weight and improving cardiovascular risk factors and cardiorespiratory fitness, which can reduce the incidence of these surgical complications. In addition, the performance of physical activity after surgery enhances its effects, generating greater reductions in total weight and cardiovascular risk factors. Furthermore, physical activity has shown to be a factor of great importance for weight maintenance, and, therefore, can be a key point to avoid recurrences in different comorbidities. Although cardiorespiratory exercise at low and moderate intensities has been classically recommended for weight loss, this trend is currently changing. In recent years, several studies have determined that performing exercise at high intensities, adding resistance training to an exercise program, generates greater losses of fat mass and reductions in cardiovascular risk factors compared to traditional recommendations.

Chapter 2 - Endothelial dysfunction is a well-described precursor to the development of clinically overt coronary and peripheral artery disease and is present early in the course of the disease. It reflects not only the global atherosclerotic status, but also the degree of rigidity of the whole artery system, thus representing an independent predictor of future CV events and all-cause mortality. The measurement of endothelial function could therefore represent an additional prognostic marker of cardiovascular risk.

The current gold standard methods to evaluate the endothelial function are intracoronary or intra-brachial infusions of vasoactive agents that enhance the release of endothelial nitric oxide (such as acetylcholine and bradykinin) and offer direct quantification of vascular response to NO. However these tests are invasive, expensive and not easily reliable.

Hence it appears clear the urge to find methods that could evaluate the endothelial function in an easier and not invasive way. In this sense various techniques have been tested in the recent past, but only two of them have shown a similar and strong correlation with cardiovascular risk compared to the invasive methods.

The more widely used is Brachial artery flow-mediated dilatation (FMD) which is based on ultrasound measures of flow-mediated changes in arterial diameter in superficial arteries (for example the brachial, radial or femoral vessels). This changes are caused by shear-stress induced generation of endothelial derived vasoactive mediators, especially represented by NO.

A more recent method is Peripheral arterial tonometry (PAT) that uses fingertip plethysmography to measure pulse volume amplitude: its changes in response to hyperemia have been shown to be nitric oxide (NO)-dependent. This suggests that PAT is a measure of endothelial function.

Despite these methods give an indirect estimate of endothelial function, the studies that evaluated FMD and PAT showed that they are independent CV risk factors and predictors of CV events and all-cause mortality. This is even more evident in the population with previously assessed CVD or with other CV risk factors.

Further research to evaluate the prognostic utility of both these methods (especially for the more recent PAT) is necessary to compare them with invasive endothelial function test in clinical practice.

Chapter 3 - The inner ear may be impaired by vascular affections since it is supplied by a terminal blood flow and has a sustained metabolic activity. It has been reported that the function of labyrinthine vessels can be influenced by several local factors such as perivascular sympathetic innervation, arterial systemic blood pressure and labyrinth liquids pressure ratio, antidiuretic hormone receptors, endothelial dysfunction and ionic transport mechanisms.

A possible link between microvascular inner ear disease and sudden sensorineural hearing loss (SSNHL) has been proposed: a sudden labyrinth oxygen lack may be responsible for acute inner ear damage, involving hair cells and then affecting hearing or vestibular function. Moreover, a primary autonomic vascular dysregulation has been related to acute cochlear damage. Many Authors have investigated the possible involvement of cardiovascular risk factors (i.e., hypertension, diabetes mellitus, hypercholesterolemia, hyperhomocysteinemia) in the pathogenesis of sudden sensorineural hearing loss. Furthermore, microcirculation defects, frequently associated to atherosclerosis, have been reported to play a major role in the onset of acute cochlear damage.

The aim of this chapter is to review the relationship between cardiovascular risk factors, systemic circulatory diseases and inner ear disorders, particularly focusing on the involvement of cardiovascular factors in the pathogenesis of SSNHL.

Chapter 4 - Impaired glucose tolerance, hypertension, and dyslipidemia have been described as metabolic syndrome (MetS). MetS is associated with an increased cardiovascular risk. A close association between morbid obesity and MetS has been highlighted in several clinical studies. Disease risk increases with increasing body mass index (BMI). However, BMI can be misleading for certain body constitutions. Thus, other parameters have been proposed as predictors of cardiovascular risk. Among them, the adiposity, the Framingham Index and the Atherogenic Index (Triglycerids/HDL-c.).

Bariatric surgery has been shown to be effective in achieving and maintaining weight change and reducing obesity-related comorbidities. Malabsorptive procedures (biliopancreatic diversion and duodenal switch) have been associated with the greatest reduction of cardiovascular risk, associated with a greatest improvement in obesity-related comorbidities (diabetes mellitus, hypertension and dyslipidemia). On the other hand, the lowest improvement is obtained after restrictive procedures (Adjustable gastric banding (AGB). However, despite sleeve gastrectomy is also considered a restrictive procedure, the reported improvement of cardiovascular risk reduction is greater than after AGB, as a certain hormonal effect is also involved in this technique-

In this chapter the authors will review the current evidence of obesity-related comorbidities and cardiovascular risk factor index after different bariatric approaches.

Chapter 5 - Cardiovascular diseases (CVD) are the leading cause of death in both men and women. There has been steady decline in mortality from CVD in middle-aged men (35 to 54 years) based on recent data from the National Health and Nutrition Examination Surveys (NHANES) but for women this rate has remained relatively unchanged. Although there are similarities in most classic risk factors in men and women, there are varying implications of these risk factors for both genders. Because of higher proportion of women in aging population with higher expression of cardiovascular risk factors, each year more women than men die because of CVD. There is increased prevalence of risk factors for heart disease in women such as obesity, smoking and diabetes and it is likely responsible for increasing burden of heart disease in women of young age. This increased risk is often under recognized because of misperception of protective effect of female hormones. Clear sex differences have been described in the epidemiology, pathophysiology, clinical presentation of disease, prevalence of risk factors and response to diagnostic tests. Furthermore, several risk factors that solely affect women include oral contraceptives, hormone replacement therapy, pregnancy-related heart disease and menopausal status. Females are also significantly under represented in cardiovascular clinical trials. Newer studies have noted marked sex difference in cardiovascular outcomes in preventive strategies and effects of therapy.

In spite of the growing evidence of magnitude of heart disease in women, they are still evaluated less intensively; risk is often undermined, under referred for diagnostic testing and not treated as aggressively as men. Increasing awareness and identification of gender based differences in cardiovascular risk factors needs more attention, which should result in a better primary and secondary prevention of cardiovascular events.

In: A Closer Look at Cardiovascular … ISBN: 978-1-53613-939-6
Editor: Faris van Kilsdonk

Chapter 1

THE EFFECTS OF EXERCISE PROGRAMS ON CARDIOVASCULAR RISK FACTORS IN PATIENTS UNDERGOING BARIATRIC SURGERY

Artur Marc Hernández[1], PhD and Jaime Ruiz-Tovar[2], MD, PhD

[1]Laboratory of Training Analysis and Optimization, Sports Research Center, Miguel Hernández University, Elche, Alicante, Spain

[2]Department of Surgery, University Hospital Rey Juan Carlos, Mostoles, Madrid, Spain

ABSTRACT

In recent decades, obesity levels have increased worldwide, increasing the prevalence of morbid obesity. This type of obesity is associated with a large number of comorbidities that increase the mortality risk of the patients who suffer it. Therefore, it is necessary to apply a treatment to this type of population. Bariatric surgery has proven to be an effective method, generating large weight reductions and improving cardiovascular risk factors, thus increasing the life expectancy of patients who undergo it. However, this surgery has certain disadvantages. On the one hand, some factors, such as total weight, comorbidities associated with obesity or low cardiorespiratory fitness, are associated with a greater number of surgical complications and a higher rate of intra and postoperative mortality. On the other hand, one of the most common problems after surgery is the weight regain, which is associated with a relapse in different comorbidities, such as diabetes mellitus.

Physical activity has been proved to be an effective tool for reducing total weight and improving cardiovascular risk factors and cardiorespiratory fitness, which can reduce the incidence of these surgical complications. In addition, the performance of physical activity after surgery enhances its effects, generating greater reductions in total weight and cardiovascular risk factors. Furthermore, physical activity has shown to be a factor of great importance for weight maintenance, and, therefore, can be a key point to avoid recurrences in different comorbidities. Although cardiorespiratory exercise at low and moderate intensities has been classically recommended for weight loss, this trend is currently changing. In recent years, several studies have determined that performing exercise at high intensities, adding resistance training to an exercise program, generates greater losses of fat mass and reductions in cardiovascular risk factors compared to traditional recommendations.

1. Introduction

Definition of Obesity, Resting Metabolic Rate and Body Tissues

Obesity is defined as an excess of fat mass that is associated with high risks for health [1]. This excess of fat mass occurs due to a prolonged state under a positive energy balance, that is, when energy intake is greater than daily energy expenditure. There are 3 components that will determine this daily energy expenditure [2]:

1. *Thermic effect of feeding*: this concept refers to the energy expenditure that is produced by the ingestion of food. It is the energy consumed in digesting, absorbing, using and storing nutrients [3]. This energy cost is different for each macronutrient, being very low for fats (0-3%), medium for carbohydrates (5-10%)

and higher for proteins (20-30%) (4). It contributes around 10% to the daily energy expenditure [2].

2. *Thermic effect of activity*: refers to the energy consumed due to physical activity (PA), therefore, it is a factor that varies greatly depending on individuals. It is especially important, because it is directly related to the activity performed, hence it has influence the basal metabolic rate (RMR). For example, PA can increase the FFM, in this way generates an increase in the RMR [5]. It has been reported that this component contributes between 15-30% to daily energy expenditure [2].
3. *Resting metabolic rate*: is the energy consumed by the body for maintaining physiological functions (body temperature, breathing, and other vital functions). It can be a key factor in controlling obesity, since it is the component that contributes the most to daily energy expenditure (60-75%) [2]. It is mainly determined by the FFM [6].

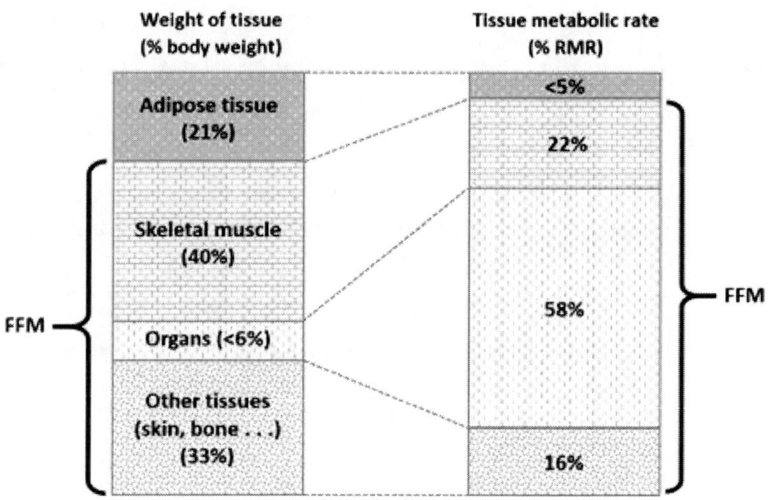

Figure 1. Distribution of body tissues and contribution of each tissue to the resting metabolic rate. Adapted from Dullo et al. [11].
Abbreviations: RMR, resting metabolic rate; FFM, fat free mass.

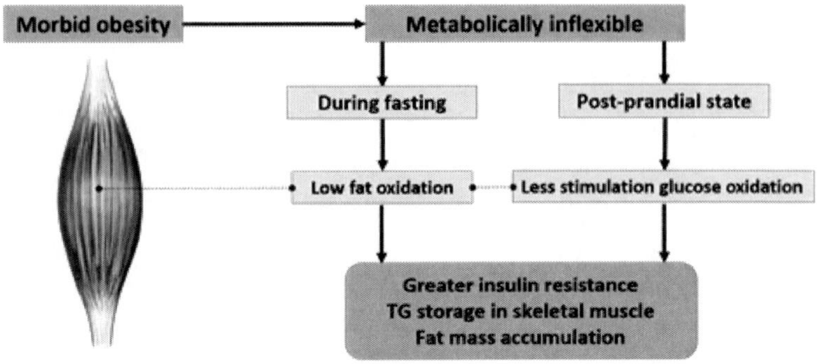

Figure 2. Skeletal muscle metabolism in patients with morbid obesity. Adapted of kelley et al. [229].

The body is integrated of different tissues. It is distinguished between adipose tissue and fat-free mass, which is composed by organs, other tissues such as skin or bones, and skeletal muscle (Figure 1). The latter is of great importance, and in recent decades has been recognized as a powerful endocrine organ [7, 8]. Among other aspects, skeletal muscle is responsible for eliminating approximately 75% of glucose after meal [9], and has an important storage function, since 80% of the body's glycogen is stored in it [10]. On the other hand, it consumes a large amount of energy at rest, about 22% of the RMR [11], which comes mainly from the oxidation of fatty acids [12]. However, in obese patients, especially in subjects with morbid obesity, it has been seen that those functions are damaged, and they are metabolically inflexible. That is, during fasting they have a low capacity to fat oxidation, which can be 58% lower than in lean subjects [13], and in a postprandial state have a lower oxidation of glucose. This will cause greater insulin resistance, storage of triglycerides in the muscle and accumulation of fat mass (Figure 2) [9, 14].

Obesity Prevalence

Progress has led to changes in society that have generated an obesogenic environment. On the one hand, the mechanization of industries and the emergence of computers have contributed to a decrease in PA at work, and an increase in sedentary jobs [15]. In addition, new forms of leisure and transportation have appeared, which are more sedentary, such as the television or the use of the car. All this causes that the levels of PA of the population have greatly decreased. For example, in the United States, PA levels decreased from 235.2 MET-hours/week in 1965 to 159.5 MET-hours/week in 2009 [16]. On the other hand, economic development and global trade liberalization have provoked changes in dietary patterns [17], where the "Western diet" has been imposed, which is a type of diet characterized by high intake of fat, added sugars, refined carbohydrates and animal-source foods [18]. In addition, energy intake in the world has increased from 2358 Kcal/day/capita to 2803 Kcal/day/capita between 1964 and 1999 [19].

These factors have led to the fact that, in recent decades, obesity levels have increased greatly in all regions of the world [20, 21].

From 572 million people with overweight or obesity in 1980, it has been estimated an increase to 1.46 billion in 2008, of which 508 million were obese [22]. While other studies concluded that in 2015 there were 603.7 million people with obesity [23]. And the forecasts are not positive, if the trend continues, it is estimated that in the year 2030, 57.8% of the world population will suffer from obesity or overweight, and 19.7% will be obese [24].

However, the problem is even greater, since levels of morbid obesity (Body Mass Index (BMI) ≥ 40 kg·m^{-2}) are also increasing acutely. Different countries show relative raises in morbid obesity of between 33-200% [25–27]. For instance, in Australia, morbid obesity increased from 1.4% to 3.1% between 1995 and 2012 [28], in Canada, it increased from 0.3% registered in 1985 to 1.6% in 2011 [29], while in the United States this increase was from 0.9% to 3.5% between 1990 and 2008 [30]. It is estimated that, if this trend continues, morbid obesity will affect 6% of men and 9% of women of the world's population in the year 2025 [31].

These high levels of obesity generate great health risks. It has been widely reported that excess weight is a determining factor in the development of type 2 diabetes mellitus [32], hypertension [33], hyperlipidemia [34] and cardiovascular risk [35]. Particularly, above all, this risk is greater with a higher BMI. Subjects with a BMI greater than 35 $kg \cdot m^{-2}$ have a risk 42.1 times higher than subjects with a normal weight [36]. Furthermore, 51.3% of subjects with morbid obesity suffer from hypertension, meanwhile 62.5% suffer from dyslipidemia [34]. All these factors contribute to the fact that obesity is directly associated with mortality (Figure 3) [37, 38]. Indeed, a high BMI caused 4 million deaths worldwide in 2015, of which, about 70% were due to cardiovascular disease [23]. In addition, the risk of mortality increases with the BMI, with a hazard ratio of 1.45 for class I obesity and 2.76 for class III obesity [39].

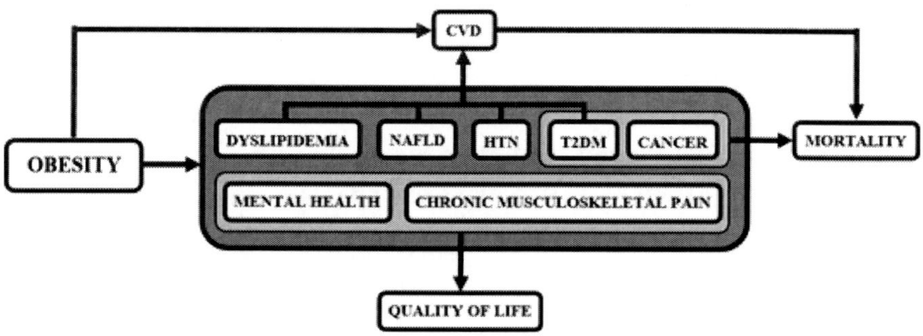

Figure 3. Most common health consequences caused by obesity.
Abbreviations: CVD, cardiovascular disease; NAFLD, nonalcoholic fatty liver disease; HTN, hypertension; T2DM, type 2 diabetes mellitus.

These aspects show the need to reduce the obesity levels of the population. Normally, through of the use of drugs, diet and PA, reductions in the body weight of obese patients are achieved [40]. But in extreme cases, such as morbid obesity, sometimes these methods are not enough [41], and an effective alternative is bariatric surgery (BS).

Bariatric Surgery

Bariatric surgery is a surgical procedure that consists of a reduction in the capacity of food intake (intragastric balloon, vertical banded gastroplasty etc.), a decrease in the absorption capacity of nutrients (biliopancreatic diversion), or well, in a combination of both (gastric bypass) [42, 43]. This surgery is performed on individuals with a BMI $\geq$ 40 kg·m^{-2} or whit a BMI $\geq$ 35 kg·m^{-2} associated with some comorbidity, such as diabetes, hypertension or obstructive sleep apnea (OSA) [44].

The first surgery was performed in Sweden in 1952, by Viktor Henrikson, and it was malabsorptive type [45]. This was followed by a process of development of the surgery, giving rise to the first mixed surgery (gastric bypass) in 1966, and to the first restrictive surgery in 1971, both performed by Edward E. Mason [46]. From this point, BS has evolved, until now it is considered one of the most effective treatments for morbid obesity [47]. In fact, in recent decades, the number of surgeries has increased in parallel with the increase of morbid obesity. In only 16 years (between 1997-2013) the number of surgeries has raised from 40,000 to 468,609 worldwide (Figure 4) [47]. Currently, of all these surgeries performed, the most frequently performed surgical techniques are sleeve gastrectomy and gastric bypass [47], the latter being considered the gold standard of surgery for obesity [48].

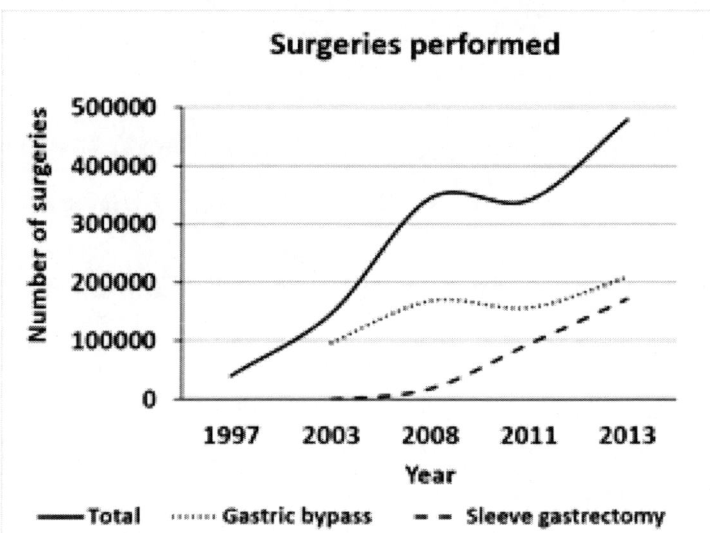

Figure 4. Evolution bariatric surgery.

Sarcopenic Obesity

Sarcopenic obesity refers to a disproportion between the amount of lean mass and fat mass, in which the fat mass exceeds the weight that lean mass could support [49]. It has a multifactorial origin. On the one hand, sarcopenic obesity is reached when the total weight is increased at the expense of an increase in fat mass. On the other hand, it is reached when, for example, subjects with morbid obesity lose a large amount of weight, with a large decrease in FFM, but they are still obese subjects [50], which is common in bariatric patients.

This sarcopenic obesity causes certain disadvantages. On the one hand, subjects with sarcopenic obesity may have impaired functional capacity [49]. On the other hand, the loss of FFM can lead to a decrease in the RMR, and therefore, induce an increase in fat mass [51]. Last, sarcopenic obesity influences in the cardiometabolic health of the patients. Subjects suffering from sarcopenic obesity have higher levels of blood pressure and greater insulin resistance than subjects with obesity or sarcopenia, as well as an increased risk of developing diabetes mellitus [52, 53]. As a result of all this, sarcopenic obesity increases the risk of suffering cardiovascular disease and mortality risk, which is higher compared to subjects who are only obese or sarcopenic [52, 54, 55].

2. Exercise Before Bariatric Surgery

Cardiovascular Risk Factors and Operative Complications

Normally, patients who are waiting for BS usually suffer from different comorbidities. Among others, it has been reported that 34-54.9% suffer from hypertension, 22-44.8% of OSA, 18-33.7% have type 2 diabetes mellitus and 7.4-50.2% of dyslipidemia [56–58]. On the one hand, this comorbidities such as hypertension, diabetes and hyperlipidemia are associated with mortality at 30 days after surgery [59–61]. On the other hand, these contribute to increase the risk of suffering post-operative complications. In a recent study, it is shown that 48% of patients who suffered postoperative complications had hypertension, and 30% had dyslipidemia [62]. In addition, hypertension and hyperlipidemia are shown as predictors of postoperative complications [62]. While in other studies, it is noticed that 52.9% of patients with diabetes and 57.6% of patients with OSA suffered moderate complications after surgery [63]. In turn, the preoperative weight is also a predictor of mortality and complications of surgery [61, 64], showing a greater risk of mortality with an increase in body mass index [65].

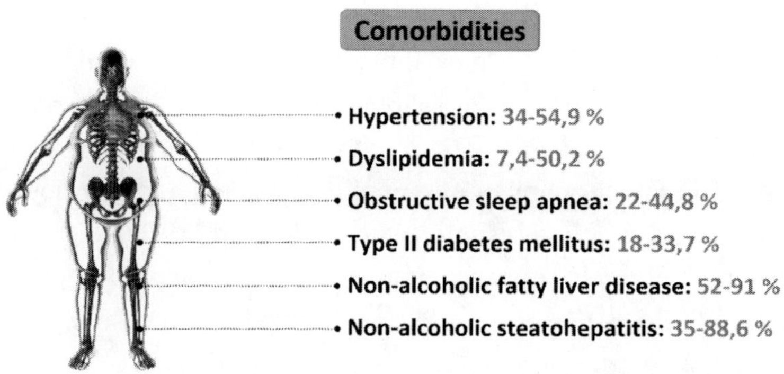

Figure 5. Percentage of subjects with specific comorbidities in patients waiting for bariatric surgery.

Along with this, it has been reported that between 52% and 91% of patients awaiting BS have non-alcoholic fatty liver disease, while between 35% and 88.6% suffer from non-alcoholic steatohepatitis [66–70]. These liver diseases, together with high levels of visceral fat can cause certain disadvantages and complicate the surgical process. On the one hand, deposits of fat tissue in the liver turn it into a more fragile organ. Which increases the risk of injury and hemorrhage due to surgical manipulation [71, 72]. On the other hand, a greater hepatic volume, especially a greater volume of the left liver lobe, difficult the approach to the gastroesophageal junction and the visualization of top portion of the stomach and the retroesophageal area [71, 73]. In fact, in gastric bypass, a larger size of the liver has been shown to be the main responsible for the conversion of laparoscopy to open surgery in 48% of cases, while steatohepatitis is a predictor of this conversion [74, 75].

In addition to comorbidities, the functional status of patients also contributes to an increased risk of morbidity/mortality, showing that subjects who are dependent or partially dependent have a greater risk of suffering complications in the surgical process [59, 76–78]. This suggests that physical fitness level at the time of the operation may be relevant, although unfortunately, there are few data on this subject in bariatric patients. In mixed intra-abdominal surgical procedures, it has been shown that an anaerobic threshold <11 ml·kg^{-1}·min^{-1} show a cardiovascular mortality ratio of 18%, however, when the anaerobic threshold is ≥ 11 ml·kg^{-1}·min^{-1}, the mortality ratio decrease until 0.8% [79]. Furthermore, an anaerobic threshold <10.1 ml·kg^{-1}·min^{-1} predicts the number of complications [80]. In bariatric surgery, one study reported that patients with a greater number of complications, and a longer hospital stay, have a lower anaerobic threshold (with a mean of 9.9 ml·kg^{-1}·min^{-1}) [81]. While in another study, it was concluded that patients with a peak oxygen consumption of less than 15.8 ml·kg^{-1}·min^{-1} had a greater risk of suffering post-operative complications [82].

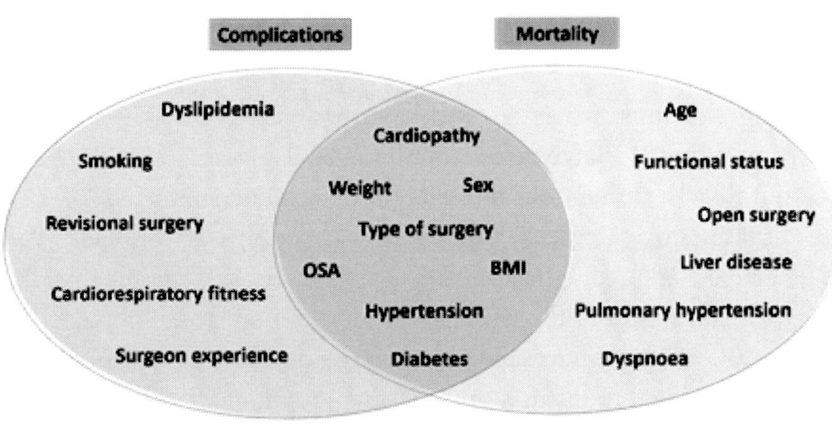

Figure 6. Factors that influence in the complications and in mortality of bariatric surgery.

All of these comorbidities associated with morbid obesity increase the risk of suffering complications, in fact, their effects are added up, since it has been shown that the greater the number of morbidities in a patient, the greater the risk of mortality [76, 77]. Consequently, surgery is not risk-free. In a meta-analysis conducted in 2014 that included 16,156 patients undergoing BS, complications were found in 17% of the surgeries performed, being 13% for sleeve gastrectomy, and 21% for gastric bypass [83]. This same study showed a perioperative mortality rate of 0.08% and a postoperative mortality of 0.31% [83].

To sum up, patients awaiting BS are associated with a high number of comorbidities. This, together with a very high weight, an inadequate functional status and a low physical condition, increase the risk of mortality and of suffering intra and postoperative complications. In addition, aspects such as a large liver size, a fatty liver, and a large amount of visceral fat, hinder the surgical process. Therefore, strategies must be pursue to maximize weight loss, reduce the number of comorbidities and increase the physical fitness in patients awaiting BS. The achievement of these objectives could increase the safety of patients and facilitate surgery. Both factors would allow to reduce the number of intra and postoperative complications, and reduce the time of the operation and the stay at the hospital, thus reducing the costs associated with the BS.

Usual Care before Surgery

Normally, in order to decrease these comorbidities associated with obesity and, thereby, decline the number of complications and the operative mortality rate, it is recommended to reduce the weight prior to surgery. This can have great advantages. On the one hand, it can reduce liver size between 5.3-18.7%, between 25.5-40% of the fat tissue deposited in the liver and approximately 17% of visceral fat [71, 84–86]. This can lead to a decrease in the duration of surgery [48, 73, 87], the number of intra and postoperative complications [48, 87–90] and generate a shorter hospital stay after surgery [87]. For this reason, many centers use restrictive or very restrictive diets in a period between 2-6 weeks prior to surgery. However, highly restrictive diets may cause the body shift into a catabolic state, producing that, a great part of the weight loss may be due to the loss of FFM, which can be approximately 40% of it [91]. This loss of FFM can lead to sarcopenic obesity [50], a state linked to a low functional capacity [51], a reduced RMR [92, 93] and an increase in insulin resistance [53]. Therefore, strategies should be applied that are able to provoke fat mass loss, maintenance FFM and generate a reduction in the comorbidities associated with obesity. Exercise can be an effective tool for this surgery.

It has been widely demonstrated that the addition of an exercise program to a nutritional intervention generates greater reductions in weight, fat mass and visceral fat compared to use a nutritional intervention in isolation [94–97], avoiding also FFM loss [96, 98]. Similarly, exercise by itself has shown to be effective both in achieving reductions in both visceral fat and fat deposited in the liver [97, 99, 100], aspects that, as we have seen, could facilitate the surgical process. At the same time, the implementation of an exercise program has been reported to be useful in achieving reductions in blood pressure, diabetes and waist circumference levels [101–103], as well as improvements in OSA [104, 105], which, could help to reduce the risk of suffering intra and postoperative complications. While, in turn, exercise is one of the most effective methods to obtain improvements in the functional capacity and cardiorespiratory fitness of individuals, which, as we have seen, are powerful predictors of surgical risk.

Physical Activity Levels in Patients Awaiting Bariatric Surgery

Despite the benefits that PA entails, patients awaiting BS show very low levels. Some studies have reported that 90% of patients are sedentary [106], while in others it is shown that candidates for bariatric surgery spend approximately 80% of the time in sedentary behaviors [107]. In fact, if you compare the levels of PA between subjects with a normal weight, and patients waiting for surgery, it is observed that only ~13% of the subjects in a normal weight do not perform moderate or vigorous PA, while this figure rises to ~68% in patients awaiting BS [108].

Therefore, it can be considered that very few of the patients have a healthy lifestyle. Studies have shown that only 4.5% of patients awaiting surgery meet the weekly recommendations for PA (≥150 min/week). Although other studies report higher percentages, only 20% of the candidates are considered active or very active (109), or perform some type of PA [110]. However, of this PA that is performed, the one that is carried out largely is walking, between 44% and 95% of the total time allocated to the activity, followed by other activities such as gardening or playing with children [109, 111]. These activities do not include resistance training, and are made at low intensities. So, we should ask ourselves if the PA that bariatric patients perform is adequate to generate fat mass losses and health benefits.

Exercise in Patients Awaiting Bariatric Surgery

Unfortunately, currently, there is a few research in which the effects of exercise have been studied in patients awaiting BS. Most studies in which an exercise program has been applied, have shown reductions in the total weight of the subjects who participated. On the one and, a resistance training generates reductions of between 1.41-7.5% total weight, from 5.3-12.5% fat mass and between 3.86-7.8% waist circumference [112–115]. On the other hand, the realization of an exercise program that combines aerobic and resistance training, of 8 or 12 weeks duration, has shown to achieve reductions of weight, fat mass and visceral fat, with a maintenance of fat-free mass [116, 117]. In turn, a training program that included only aerobic exercise at low intensities also generated reductions in the total weight of the patients [118]. Besides, one aspect of great importance that many of the studies have in common is that there is an improvement in physical fitness, especially in the cardiorespiratory fitness [112, 114–117, 119, 120].

If the number of studies in patients awaiting BS is low, the quantity of studies examining the effects of exercise on cardiovascular risk factors (CVRF) in this population is still lower. However, in these studies there is a trend of exercise to improve CVRF. For example, a resistance training after surgery, that consisted of 3 series per exercise of 60 seconds to muscle failure, performed 3 times a week for 12 or 16 weeks, generated reductions in blood glucose of ~10% [114, 115], and showed a tendency to decrease the levels of total cholesterol (8.1%), LDL (-6.3%) and TG (-7.6%) [112].

Aerobic training has also proven to be an effective tool. In a 6-month study, patients were given a supervised training session a week in which 30 minutes of low-intensity aerobic exercise was performed and they were encouraged to do this in their homes. The results of this study showed reductions in total cholesterol, LDL cholesterol, triglycerides, blood glucose and blood pressure, resulting a great reduction of the CVR (-4.4 units) [118]. In another study, a program of PA focused on AT, 2 days per week for 4 months, was added to the usual care, besides subjects were encouraged to increase the number of steps walked every day. This patients had reductions in CVRF, which caused a decrease in cardiovascular risk (-3.4 units), while the control group did not show any improvement. On the contrary, it had an increase in blood glucose and triglycerides [120]. In addition, shorter training programs can also generate certain benefits. By only 7 days performing a 60 minutes of aerobic training at 65% of maximum oxygen consumption has been reduced fasting insulin concentrations and the insulin area under the curve during the oral glucose tolerance test, what indicates that there has been an improvement in the action of insulin [121].

Although there are few studies in the literature, these studies show potential benefits in patients who perform exercise before surgery. On the one hand, exercise causes reductions in weight and in comorbidities associated with obesity, while it increases in cardiorespiratory fitness, which could greatly help to reduce operative complications and hospital stay after BS. On the other hand, decreases in waist circumference indicate that visceral fat is also being reduced, thus facilitating the surgical process.

Therefore, the health system should seriously consider the inclusion of exercise programs prior to surgery.

3. Exercise in Patients Undergoing Bariatric Surgery (Short-Term)

Benefits and Disadvantages of Bariatric Surgery in the Short-Term

It has been widely argued that BS generates great benefits. In the short-term, BS causes large weight losses, causing reductions of between 20-35 kg three months after the intervention [122–124], and between approximately 35-50 kg a year after surgery, reducing to a great extent fat mass [125–127], and visceral fat [128]. Furthermore, after BS, decreases in liver volume and fatty liver levels are also generated [129, 130]. Along with this, improvements in CVRF have also been widely reported, such as decreases in resting blood pressure, glycosylated hemoglobin, LDL cholesterol, and increases in HDL cholesterol [131–133]. The results of a meta-analysis covering more than 22,000 patients showed complete remissions in 76.8% of diabetic subjects, of 61.7% of hypertensive patients, of 85.7% of patients with OSA, and a reduction of hyperlipidemia in 70% of patients [134]. All this will reduce the risk of heart disease [135, 136]. But not only physiological improvements are achieved, psychological improvements are also generated, such as increases in mental health, increased self-esteem or a decrease in depression levels [137, 138].

However, BS has, in the short-term, some disadvantages. After surgery, especially when it is malabsorptive, there is a deficiency of certain micronutrients. After gastric bypass, iron deficits have been reported in 49% of patients, of vitamin B12 in 70%, of calcium in 10%, and of Vitamin D in 50%, as well as decreases in bone mineral density [139, 140]. However, in this chapter, greater emphasis will be placed on the FFM losses. Many studies show reductions of around 10 kg of fat-free mass a year after surgery [125, 127, 141–144]. These reductions in fat-free mass can cause, among other factors, a greater insulin resistance, a decrease in the RMR and favor the accumulation of fat mass [51]. In fact, a low RMR has been associated with weight regain in bariatric patients [145–147], which is one of the most common problems in this population, as it will be seen later [110, 148–150].

Physical Activity Levels in Patients Undergoing Bariatric Surgery in the Short-Term

As seen above, most patients awaiting BS have a sedentary behavior. However, it has been widely reported that in the short-term after BS, patients increase their PA levels [151–155]. In some studies it has been shown that the percentage of patients who did not perform any PA decreased from 37.4% to 7.6% a year after surgery [156]. Other studies have reported increases between 1225 and 2749 steps/day a year after surgery [155, 157], increasing from 30% to 46% of subjects who performed at least 150 minutes of PA per week [157]. The most frequently activity performed after surgery is walking, 54.7% of patients, while only 12.7% report performing weight lifting [157]. This, as it will be seen later, may be of great importance in weight loss and the reduction of comorbidities after surgery. However, in the same way as before surgery, subjects perform little strength training, and the intensity that can be reached walking may not report the best benefits.

Exercise in Patients Undergoing Bariatric Surgery in the Short-Term

As we have seen, after surgery, a series of disadvantages are generated, which could be minimized or even avoided by performing structured exercise appropriately. Unfortunately, there are currently few studies on this, and most of them are observational studies. These studies show greater reductions in weight in subjects who perform PA after surgery [158–160], noting that only 150 minutes per week of moderate or intense PA per week are sufficient to generate greater weight losses [161]. In addition, both higher volumes and higher PA intensities performed after bariatric surgery are associated with greater weight losses [162]. However, in the short term after surgery, the important issue is not weight loss, since both patients who perform exercise and those who do not it, have large reductions in total weight. This point should focus on the FFM, although the availability of studies on this is still scarcer, since few studies analyze the effects of exercise on body composition after surgery. They have found that a greater increase in leisure time PA, was directly associated with a smaller decrease in fat-free mass [153]. While another reported that only the completion of 30 minutes 3 or more times per week showed to be effective to increase the FFM [163]. Here the volume also seems to be important, since it has been shown that the subjects who increased their steps/day more after surgery obtained skeletal muscle maintenance [164].

However, nowadays, some research has emerged on this subject. These studies show that patients who participate in a post-surgery exercise program avoid or reduce the FFM loss [165–168], although occasionally, the difference between experimental group and control group is not significant [169, 170]. In most of these studies there is only one intervention group in which an exercise program is applied, therefore, it is not established what type of exercise can be more effective after surgery. Nevertheless, one study compared a control group and two experimental groups, one of them performed only aerobic training, and the other combined aerobic and resistance training. The results showed that the group that included resistance training was the one that lost the least FFM, meanwhile the control group had the greatest reduction [168]. Therefore, although volumes and intensities are still to be determined, it seems that resistance training can be a determining factor in the maintenance of the FFM.

Avoiding the loss of FFM can be of great importance, both in the short and long term. On the one hand, as we have seen previously, the FFM (specifically the skeletal muscle) plays a fundamental role in the organism, so its maintenance could generate additional benefits to the surgery in the cardiometabolic profile of the patients, as well as a greater functional capacity. On the other hand, maintaining the FFM could prevent or minimize the reduction of RMR that is generated after surgery [171], and it has been associated with certain long-term problems, such as weight recovery [172, 173].

Although, after surgery there is an improvement in functional capacity (evaluated by the 6-minute walk test) [174], this is not the case when aerobic capacity is measured by oxygen consumption. It can be observed that in the studies that analyze oxygen consumption after surgery, there are increases when the results are normalized to the total weight of patients. Probably, these increases are due to the great weight loss that occurs, and not to an improvement in cardiorespiratory fitness, since absolute oxygen consumption does not increase [175, 176]. However, in studies in which an exercise program is applied, it can be seen how patients who perform it have greater rises in normalized oxygen consumption to weight, and increases in consumption of oxygen in absolute values [177–179]. The improvement of cardiorespiratory capacity can be of great importance in CVRF, since it is associated with a lower cardiometabolic risk [180, 181].

As previously shown, BS, by itself, generates large improvements in cardiometabolic risk factors. However, there is a proportion of patients to whom the BS fails for reducing certain comorbidities. Some authors have called these patients as resistant to bariatric surgery [182]. These patients, besides not showing improvements in cardiometabolic parameters, have lower weight losses after surgery. Although the reasons for this variability between patients are not clear yet, there are different common aspects in the "non-responsiveness to surgery," such as gender, age or preoperative weight, emphasizing an inadequate PA, since it is a factor that can be modified.

However, although the role of the exercise on CVRF remains to be determined, due to the lack of studies, it seems that it can have a positive effect. In an observational study it was obtained that, one year after surgery, total and LDL cholesterol were higher in the sedentary subjects

(<1,250 Mets/14 days), while the HDL cholesterol, although the difference was not significant, showed a tendency to be higher in active subjects (75.5 $mg{\cdot}dl^{-1}$ vs 68.6 $mg{\cdot}dl^{-1}$) [106]. Another study showed that, also one year after surgery, patients who reported an average of 96.8 minutes of aerobic exercise per week had a higher resolution of diabetes and OSA than patients who had an average of 21.1 minutes per week [183]. In addition, positive associations have been found between the number of daily steps and insulin sensitivity, and between the increase in daily minutes of PA and HDL cholesterol 9 months after surgery [184].

Recently, some experimental studies have emerged on this subject. In these studies, in the short-term (6-9 months), there are no differences between patients participating in an exercise program, and those who do not, showing all patients similar improvements in lipid profile and blood pressure levels at rest [178, 179]. However, after surgery, exercise seems to be effective in glucose metabolism. In one study, a 12-week exercise program was performed, in which 2000 kcal a week was tried to consume by aerobic exercise at 60-70% of VO_{2max} [178]. The results of this study showed a reduction in the incremental area under the curve postprandial blood glucose response in the experimental group. In turn, other studies have shown greater improvements in insulin sensitivity by performing only ~120 minutes of aerobic exercise per week, at an intensity of 60-70% [179, 185].

Although the limited availability of studies in this regard does not allow to reach a clear conclusion, it seems that the performance of aerobic exercise in the short term after surgery (6-9 months) produces additional benefits in the improvement of glycemic control. While, between 9-12 months after BS, it is observed that PA can contribute to increase HDL cholesterol, and a higher resolution of various comorbidities, such as diabetes. This seems to indicate that the use of exercise programs can help improve the cardiovascular profile in patients who do not respond adequately to surgery.

4. Exercise in Patients Undergoing Bariatric Surgery (Medium and Long-Term)

Benefits and Disadvantages of Bariatric Surgery in the Medium and Long-Term

Bariatric surgery generates diverse benefits, which decrease the risk of suffering a cardiovascular disease [135, 136], and in the long term it contributes to the fact that subjects with morbid obesity undergoing BS show an increase of approximately 7 years in their life expectancy [186].

However, one of the biggest disadvantages after BS is weight regain, which is shown above in all studies that have a follow-up period ≥5 years [187]. Weight regain occurs in a large proportion of patients (19.2% - 58.5%) [110, 148–150], and it is positively associated with the postoperative period, [110, 188] that is, the longer after surgery, greater weight regain. Therefore, it can be seen how patients decrease from 70% of EWL in the second year of surgery to 42% at 10 years. While other studies have shown that 6 years after surgery, 64% of patients had a% EWL below 50% [189].

Bariatric surgery

	Benefits	Disadvantages
Short-term	➢ Fat mass loss ➢ Improve comorbidities ➢ Improve functional capacity ➢ Quality of life increase	➢ Fat free mass loss ➢ Deficiency of micronutrients ➢ Bone mineral density decrease ➢ Resting metabolic rate decrease
Medium and long-term	➢ Cardivascular disease risk decrease ➢ Life expectancy increase	➢ Weight regain ➢ Relapse in comorbidities ➢ Revisional surgery ➢ Quality of life decrease

Figure 7. Benefits and disadvantages of bariatric surgery.

On the one hand, weight regain can lead to revisional surgery, which has been seen between 15.4% and 36% of patients [148, 150, 190]. On the other hand, weight regain can be accompanied by relapses in different comorbidities [191]. One study showed that the incidence in diabetes, hypertension and hypertriglyceridemia increased from 1% to 7%, from 24% to 41% and from 8% to 17% respectively between the 2nd and the 10th year of the surgery [192]. Similar results have been shown in the short-term, observing how the complete remission of diabetes decreased from 50.7% patients a year after surgery to 20% at 5 years, while the complete remission of the cholesterolemia decreased from 40% to 26.1% [193]. Furthermore, type 2 diabetes mellitus relapse ranges have been obtained from 19% to 35.1% of patients [194–196], and these relapses have been associated with weight regain [195, 197]. While, regarding hypertension, Benaiges et al. showed a range of relapse in 21.9% of patients between the 1st and 3rd year of surgery, with these patients showing a lower% EWL than subjects who did not relapse [198].

Physical Activity Levels in the Medium and Long-Term after Bariatric Surgery

Although there are few studies that analyze changes in PA levels in the medium and long term, it seems that over time they tend to decrease. Sjöström et al. found as the proportion of subjects who were active in leisure time and work increased after surgery, reaching a peak around the year of the same, and that from this moment began to reduce, until at 10 years, there was a great reduction in this proportion [192]. In turn, another study showed an increase in steps/day (+1526.8) and in the percentage of patients who performed 150 minutes of moderate or intense activity per week (+10.2%) two years after surgery. However, between the 2nd and the 3rd year of surgery both variables were significantly reduced (-278.9 steps/day; -7.1%, respectively) [199]. In a long-term study it was reported that at ~9 years of surgery, although 71.8% of patients reported being more active than before CB, but only 11.7% of patients performed ≥10,000 steps/day (daily recommendation), while 36.6% performed less than 5000 steps/day. In addition, 7 years after surgery, only 48% of patients reported performing ≥1 exercise session per week, while the average time spent sitting turned out to be 7.3 hours per day (200). So, it can be concluded that in the medium and long term there is a decrease in the levels of PA, there being a large proportion of patients who are not very active, and spend much of their time in sedentary behavior.

Exercise in Patients Undergoing Bariatric Surgery in the Medium and Long-Term

From our knowledge, there are few studies that investigate the role of exercise on CVRF in the medium and long term after BS. However, as we have seen above, weight control can be of great importance for CVRF, and exercise can be a fundamental tool for this. In one study, PA was evaluated 36 months after surgery, and it was found that subjects who performed between 0 and 59 minutes of aerobic exercise had an EWL of 33%, while those who performed ≥150 minutes had an EWL of 54'1%, which is considered a successful weight loss [183]. Herman et al. showed that patients who reported ≥1 weekly sessions of at least 30 minutes of moderate or vigorous exercise were more likely to maintain at least 50% of their initial weight loss (OR: 2.6), and had a lower probability of weight regain than less active subjects (OR: -3'1) [201]. In another study that modified the behavior of the patients, modifying eating habits and increasing levels of PA, it was obtained that the subjects of the experimental group had a greater weight loss at 12 months after surgery, and subsequently, they got a maintenance of the lost weight. However, subjects who did not change their habits showed a decrease in their %EWL between 12 and 36 months after surgery (from 57.5% to 49.1%) [202].

Although the majority of studies regarding this topic are observational, some experimental study has also been carried out. In one study, patients who had <50% EWL after 3 years or more of surgery were recruited. The experimental group underwent a 6-month behavioral intervention that consisted in reducing caloric intake, and in the prescription, a PA program. The results of this study showed a significant decrease in %EWL after the intervention only in the experimental group (-6.6% EWL) [203]. Last, in one study an exercise program that combined aerobic and resistance training at moderate intensities was applied in patients who had a BMI ≥ 30 between 12-24 months after surgery. The group that performed the exercise program had reductions in weight and resting blood pressure, while in the control group there was a tendency to increase weight [204].

In the studies it is observed that adding exercise to BS generates greater weight loss and that it is an effective tool to achieve weight maintenance that has been lost through surgery. In addition, exercise can be an efficient method to generate weight loss in patients with an inadequate weight loss or who suffer from weight regain.

5. Oriented New Trends Training to Health

Traditionally, to achieve weight loss in obese people, it has been recommended to perform aerobic exercise at moderate intensities, without giving much importance to the resistance, defending the volume of aerobic activity as a determining factor. While some authors stated that for achieving weight loss should be performed 5 days a week of aerobic activity, with a minimum duration of 60 minutes per session [205]. Other organizations, such as the ACSM in its position stand in 2009, proposed that performing 150-250 minutes per week of PA at moderate intensity will result in modest weight reductions, but that greater than 250 minutes per week is when the greatest benefits are achieved [206]. However, the role of resistance training on weight loss has not been given more relevance [206, 207].

Currently, this trend is changing, and it seems that there are other methods that can be more effective than aerobic training. Resistance training increases fat-free mass, and with it the RMR (208), so it can be very important both to generate weight loss and to avoid weight gain. In addition, it has been shown to be as effective in reducing CVRF as aerobic training [209]. Therefore, if resistance training is added to aerobic training, it can be an effective strategy for weight and cardiometabolic control. In recent years, research has emerged that confirms this theory. It has been found that, by combining resistance and aerobic training in the same training program, greater reductions in weight, fat mass, waist circumference and abdominal fat are achieved than through aerobic training in isolation [210–214]. Generating at the same time increases in fat-free mass [212–214]. Even the benefits of CVRF are also greater when both types of training are combined [102, 215].

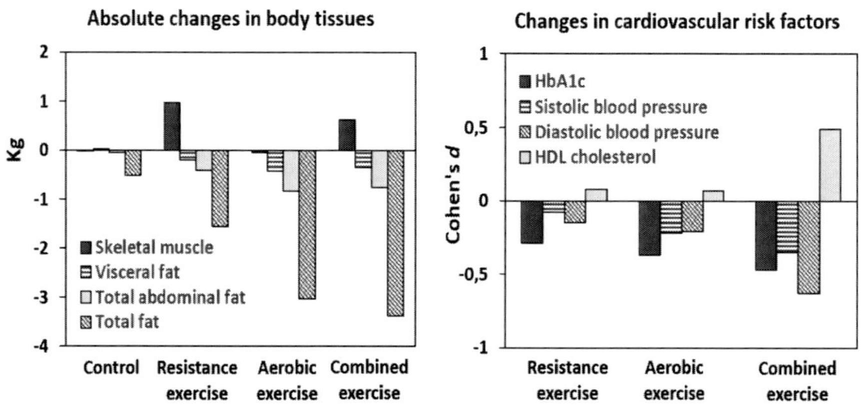

Figure 8. Impact of different exercise modalities on body tissues and cardiovascular risk factors. Dates obtained from Davidson et al. [230] and Snowling et al. [231].

On the other hand, training intensity is showing itself as a decisive component. Currently, numerous research are reporting the benefits of high intensity interval training (HIIT). HIIT is a type of exercise that combines short periods at high intensities and low intensities in the same training session, thus, when applying recovery periods, training time in more intense areas is prolonged in relation to continuous training [216]. The greater the intensity of aerobic training, the greater will be the increase in excess post-exercise oxygen consumption (EPOC) [217]. The increase in EPOC, in turn, has been related to a greater mobilization of fatty acids [218], in both healthy and obese subjects [219, 220]. This means that HIIT is an effective method to achieve fat loss as continuous training at moderate intensities [221]. Other benefits are also attributed to it, as it decreases insulin sensitivity [220, 222], reduces cholesterol [222–224], glycemia [225] and blood pressure levels [224, 226], in addition to achieving greater increases in cardiorespiratory capacity than through continuous training at moderate intensities [227]. All this results in that this type of training helps reduce the risk of suffering cardiometabolic pathologies [228].

However, one of the main advantages of HIIT is that all these results are achieved in 40% less training time than if continuous training were employed [221], which leaves more time in a training session so that other capacities can be worked on, as the strength. As we have seen previously, resistance training can provoke great benefits, but training intensity is also important. In studies with obese subjects who train at intensities between 70-80% of the repetition maximum (RM), gains of fat-free mass are obtained [212–214]. A recent review that analyzes the effects of training intensity, has concluded that the intensities that cause more favorable changes in body composition and in certain CVRF are between 75-80% of the RM for resistance training, and above 75% VO_{2max} for aerobic training, and not between 55-75%, as has been traditionally prescribed [96].

Therefore, adding an exercise program to a nutritional intervention can be an effective strategy to maximize the results in weight loss and in the improvement of CVRF. The inclusion of strength training in an exercise program can avoid reductions in FFM, while aerobic training at high intensities can, among other benefits, generate greater losses of fat mass. Consequently, for an exercise program to be as efficient as possible and generate the greatest benefits in the CVRF, it should combine both types of exercise (resistance and aerobic training), initiated at moderate intensities, but progressing to train at high intensities.

Conclusion

Exercise may be of great importance in the control of CVRF in bariatric patients. This control of the CVRF can be done in different ways.

On the one hand, exercise by itself generates improvements in glycemic control, hypertension, lipid profile and other comorbidities associated with obesity. On the other hand, when a nutritional intervention is combined with exercise, large weight losses occur, which is associated with an improvement in comorbidities.

Furthermore, it is important to notice that cardiorespiratory fitness is a very high importance for cardiovascular risk factors, and the fact of rising it is able to prevent to some degree, cardiovascular diseases. In the same way, skeletal muscle is a powerful endocrine organ that must not be forgotten. It has relevant functions such as elimination of post-prandial glucose, glucose storing or a high oxidation of fatty acids at rest. For that reason, in these patients who have a high cardiovascular risk, exercise must be aimed at the rising of cardiorespiratory fitness, maintaining skeletal muscle levels and rising muscular quality.

However, due to different disadvantages that BS can present, the objectives of the exercise should be different at each stage of the surgery. Prior to surgery, it should be sought to generate greater losses of fat mass, especially of visceral fat, and to help reduce the comorbidities associated with obesity, in addition to increasing cardiorespiratory fitness. All this will reduce the surgical risk, and can help to decrease the number of complications and mortality in these patients, as well as a shorter hospital stay, which could reduce the health cost of the operation.

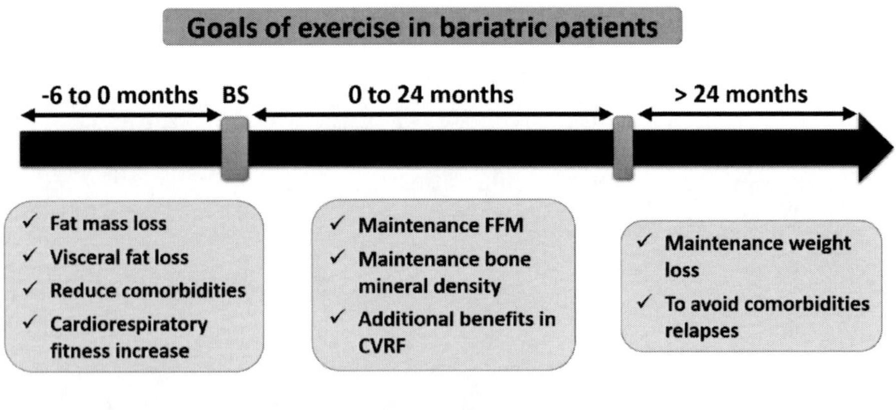

Figure 9. Exercise goals before and after bariatric surgery.

Bariatric surgery generates large losses of fat mass by itself, therefore, after surgery (especially in the first months), exercise should be oriented mainly to the maintenance of FFM, of the RMR and of the bone mineral density, for that reasons, the resistance training is fundamental. In addition, exercise can help by reducing comorbidities in patients who fail through bariatric surgery.

Normally, after BS there is a point of maximum weight loss, which is usually reached between 12-24 months after surgery. At this point, exercise should focus on maintaining the weight loss through BS. Possibly, this would be an effective strategy to avoid relapse in comorbidities that occurs in some patients, since these relapses are associated with weight regain.

REFERENCES

[1] Sellen D. Physical status: the use and interpretation of anthropometry. Report of a WHO Expert Committee. *WHO Technical Report.* 1998. p. 1–452.

[2] Poehlman E. A review: exercise and its influence on resting energy metabolism in man. *Med Sci Sport Exerc*. 1989;21(5):515–25.

[3] Pinheiro Volp AC, Esteves de Oliveira F., Duarte Moreira Alves R, Esteves E., Bressan J. Energy expenditure: components and evaluation methods. *Nutr Hosp*. 2011;26(3):430–40.

[4] Tappy L. Thermic effect of food and sympathetic nervous system activity in humans. *Reprod Nutr Dev*. 1996;36(4):391–7.

[5] Strasser B, Schobersberger W. *Evidence for Resistance Training as a Treatment Therapy in Obesity*. 2011;2011.

[6] Illner K, Brinkmann G, Heller M, Bosy-Westphal a, Müller MJ. Metabolically active components of fat free mass and resting energy expenditure in nonobese adults. *Am J Physiol Endocrinol Metab*. 2000;278(2):E308–15.

[7] Pedersen BK, Febbraio MA. Muscles, exercise and obesity: Skeletal muscle as a secretory organ. *Nat Rev Endocrinol.* Nature Publishing Group; 2012;8(8):457–65.

[8] Kim TN, Choi KM. The implications of sarcopenia and sarcopenic obesity on cardiometabolic disease. *J Cell Biochem.* 2015;116(7):1171–8.

[9] Houmard JA, Pories WJ, Dohm GL. Severe obesity: evidence for a deranged metabolic program in skeletal muscle? *Exerc Sport Sci Rev.* 2013;40(4):204–10.

[10] Jensen J, Rustad PI, Kolnes AJ, Lai YC. The role of skeletal muscle glycogen breakdown for regulation of insulin sensitivity by exercise. *Front Physiol*. 2011;2:1–11.

[11] Dulloo AG, Jacquet J, Solinas G, Montani J, Schutz Y. Body composition phenotypes in pathways to obesity and the metabolic syndrome. *Int J Obes.* Nature Publishing Group; 2010;34(S2): S4–17.

[12] Saltin B, Helge JW. Skeletal muscles, physical activity and health. *Orthopade*. 2000;29(11):941–7.

[13] Hulver MW, Berggren JR, Cortright RN, Dudek RW, Thompson RP, Pories WJ, et al. Skeletal muscle lipid metabolism with obesity. *Am J Physiol Endocrinol Metab*. 2003;284(4):E741-7.

[14] Kelley DE, Goodpaster B, Wing RR, Simoneau J a. Skeletal muscle fatty acid metabolism in association with insulin resistance, obesity, and weight loss. *Am J Physiol*. 1999;277(6 Pt 1):E1130–41.

[15] Church TS, Thomas DM, Tudor-locke C, Katzmarzyk PT, Conrad P, Rodarte RQ, et al. Trends over 5 Decades in U.S. Occupation-Related Physical Activity and Their Associations with Obesity. *PLoS One.* 2011;6(5):1–7.

[16] Ng SW, Popkin BM. Time use and physical activity: A shift away from movement across the globe. *Obes Rev*. 2012;13(8):659–80.

[17] Malik VS, Willett WC, Hu FB. Global obesity: trends, risk factors and policy implications. *Nat Rev Endocrinol.* Nature Publishing Group; 2013;9(1):13–27.

[18] Popkin BM. Nutrition Transition and the Global Diabetes Epidemic. *Curr Diab Rep*. 2015;15(9):64.

[19] Vasileska A, Rechkoska G. Global and Regional Food Consumption Patterns and Trends. *Procedia-Social Behav Sci* [Internet]. 2012;44:363–9.

[20] Prentice A, Ph D, Jebb S, Ph D. Energy Intake/Physical Activity Interactions in the Homeostasis of Body Weight Regulation. *Nutr Rev.* 2004;62(7):S98-104.

[21] Ng M, Fleming T, Robinson M, Thomson B, Graetz N, Margono C, et al. Global, regional, and national prevalence of overweight and obesity in children and adults during 1980–2013: a systematic analysis for the Global Burden of Disease Study 2013. *Lancet.* 2014;384(9945):766–81.

[22] Stevens GA, Singh GM, Lu Y, Danaei G, Lin JK, Finucane MM, et al. National, regional, and global trends in adult overweight and obesity prevalences. *Popul Health Metr*. 2012; 10 (1) 1–16.

[23] GBD 2015 Obesity Collaborators. Health Effects of Overweight and Obesity in 195 Countries over 25 Years. *N Engl J Med.* 2017;377(1):1–15.

[24] Kelly T, Yang W, Chen C-S, Reynolds K, He J. Global burden of obesity in 2005 and projections to 2030. *Int J Obes*. 2008;32(9):1431–7.

[25] Lear SA, Wu CH. Prevalence and trends of adult obesity in the US, 1999-2012. *ISRN Obes*. 2014;2014:1–6.

[26] Sturm R, Hattori A. Morbid obesity rates continue to rise rapidly in the United States. *Int J Obes* (Lond). 2013;37(6):889–91.

[27] Basterra-Gortari FJ, Beunza JJ, Bes-Rastrollo M, Toledo E, García-López M, Martínez-González MA. Increasing trend in the prevalence of morbid obesity in Spain: from 1.8 to 6.1 per thousand in 14 years. *Rev española Cardiol.* 2011;64(5):424–6.

[28] Keating C, Backholer K, Gearon E, Stevenson C, Swinburn B, Moodie M, et al. Prevalence of class-I, class-II and class-III obesity in Australian adults between 1995 and 2011-12. *Obes Res Clin Pract*. 2015;9(6):553–62.

[29] Twells LK, Gregory DM, Reddigan J, Midodzi WK. Current and predicted prevalence of obesity in Canada: a trend analysis. *C open.* 2014;2(1):E18-26.

[30] Finkelstein EA, Khavjou OA, Thompson H, Trogdon JG, Pan L, Sherry B. Obesity and Severe Obesity Forecasts Through 2030. *Am J Prev Med*. 2012;42(6):563–70.

[31] NCD Risk Factor Collaboration. Trends in adult body-mass index in 200 countries from 1975 to 2014: a pooled analysis of 1698 population-based measurement studies with 19·2 million participants. *Lancet*. NCD Risk Factor Collaboration. Open Access article distributed under the terms of CC BY; 2016;387 (10026):1377–96.

[32] Hu F, Manson J, Stampfer M, Colditz G, Liu S, Solomon C, et al. Diet, lifestyle, and the risk of type 2 diabetes mellitus in women. *N Engl J Med*. 2001;345(11):790–7.

[33] Brown CD, Higgins M, Donato KA, Rohde FC, Garrison R, Obarzanek E, et al. Body mass index and the prevalence of hypertension and dyslipidemia. *Obes Res*. 2000;8(9):605–19.

[34] Bays HE, Toth PP, Kris-Etherton PM, Abate N, Aronne LJ, Brown WV, et al. Obesity, adiposity, and dyslipidemia: A consensus statement from the National Lipid Association. *J Clin Lipidol*. 2013;7(4):304–83.

[35] Fock KM, Khoo J. Diet and exercise in management of obesity and overweight. *J Gastroenterol Hepatol.* 2013;28(Suppl 4):59–63.

[36] Chan JM, Rimm EB, Colditz GA, Stampfer MJ, Willett WC. Obesity, Fat Distribution, and Weight Gain as Risk Factors for Clinical Diabetes in Men. *Diabtes Care*. 1994;17(9):961–9.

[37] Patel A V, Hildebrand JS, Gapstur SM. Body Mass Index and All-Cause Mortality in a Large Prospective Cohort of White and Black U.S. Adults. *PLoS One*. 2014;9(10):e109153.

[38] Flegal KM, Graubard BI, Williamson DF, Gail MH. Cause-specific excess deaths associated with underweight, overweight, and obesity. *Jama.* 2007;298(17):2028–37.

[39] The Global Mortality Colaboration TGM. Body-mass index and all-cause mortality: individual-participant-data meta-analysis of 239 prospective studies in four continents. *Lancet.* 2016;388(10046): 776–86.

[40] Avenell a, Broom J, Brown TJ, Poobalan a, Aucott L, Stearns SC, et al. Systematic review of the long-term effects and economic consequences of treatments for obesity and implications for health improvement. *Health Technol Assess*. 2004;8(21):iii–iv, 1-182.

[41] Rubio M, Martínez C, Vidal O. Documento de consenso sobre cirugía bariátrica. *Rev Esp Obes*. 2004;4:223–49.

[42] Sasaki A, Wakabayashi G, Yonei Y. Current status of bariatric surgery in Japan and effectiveness in obesity and diabetes. *J Gastroenterol*. 2014;49(1):57–63.

[43] Jaunoo S, Southall P. Bariatric surgery. *Obes Surg*. 2010;8(2):86–9.

[44] Khwaja HA, Bonanomi G. Bariatric surgery: techniques, outcomes and complications. *Curr Anaesth Crit Care*. 2010;21(1):31–8.

[45] Baker MT. The History and Evolution of Bariatric Surgical Procedures. *Surg Clin North Am*.2011;91(6):1181–201.

[46] González-gonzález JJ, Sanz-álvarez L, García C. La obesidad en la historia de la cirugía. [Obesity in the history of surgery.] *Cir Esp*. 2008;84(4):188–95.

[47] Angrisani L, Santonicola A, Iovino P, Formisano G, Buchwald H, Scopinaro N. Bariatric Surgery Worldwide 2013. *Obes Surg*. 2015;25(10):1822–32.

[48] Blackburn GL, Hutter MM, Harvey AM, Apovian CM, Boulton HRW, Cummings S, et al. Expert panel on weight loss surgery: executive report update. *Obesity* (Silver Spring). 2009; 17(5): 842–62.

[49] Cauley JA. An Overview of Sarcopenic Obesity. *J Clin Densitom*. 2015;18(4):499–505.

[50] Prado CMM, Wells JCK, Smith SR, Stephan BCM, Siervo M. Sarcopenic obesity: A Critical appraisal of the current evidence. *Clin Nutr*.2012;31(5):583–601.

[51] Parr EB, Coffey VG, Hawley JA. "Sarcobesity": A metabolic conundrum. *Maturitas*.2013;74(2):109–13.

[52] Curvello-silva K, Barreto-medeiros JM. Association between sarcopenic obesity and cardiovascular risk : where are we ? *Nutr Hosp*. 2016;33(5):1245–55.

[53] Srikanthan P, Hevener AL, Karlamangla AS. Sarcopenia exacerbates obesity-associated insulin resistance and dysglycemia: Findings from the national health and nutrition examination survey III. *PLoS One*. 2010;5(5).

[54] Kim J-H, Cho JJ, Park YS. Relationship between Sarcopenic Obesity and Cardiovascular Disease Risk as Estimated by the Framingham Risk Score. *J Korean Med Sci*. 2015;30(3):264–71.

[55] Wannamethee SG, Atkins JL. Muscle loss and obesity: the health implications of sarcopenia and sarcopenic obesity. *Proc Nutr Soc*. 2015;(December 2014):1–8.

[56] Livingston EH. Procedure incidence and in-hospital complication rates of bariatric surgery in the United States. *Am J Surg*. 2004;188(2):105–10.

[57] Goergen M, Arapis K, Limgba A, Schiltz M, Lens V, Azagra JS. Laparoscopic Roux-en-Y gastric bypass versus laparoscopic vertical banded gastroplasty : results of a 2-year follow-up study. *Surg Endosc*. 2007;21(4):659–64.

[58] Jonathan F, Kole KL, Yenumula PR, English WJ. Predicting Risk for Serious Complications With Bariatric Surgery Results from the Michigan Bariatric Surgery Collaborative. *Ann Surg*. 2011;254(4):633–40.

[59] Benotti P, Wood GC, Winegar DA, Petrick AT, Still CD, Argyropoulos G, et al. Risk factors associated with mortality after Roux-en-Y gastric bypass surgery. *Ann Surg*. 2014;259(1):123–30.

[60] Nguyen NT, Nguyen B, Smith B, Reavis KM, Elliott C, Hohmann S. Proposal for a bariatric mortality risk classification system for patients undergoing bariatric surgery. *Surg Obes Relat Dis*. 2013;9(2):239–46.

[61] Fernandez AZ, Demaria EJ, Tichansky DS, Kellum JM, Wolfe LG, Meador J, et al. Experience with over 3,000 open and laparoscopic bariatric procedures. *Surg Endosc*. 2004;18(2):193–7.

[62] Coblijn UK, Karres J, Raaff CAL De, Castro SMM De, Lagarde SM, Tets WF Van, et al. Predicting postoperative complications after bariatric surgery : the Bariatric Surgery Index for Complications, BASIC. *Surg Endosc*. Springer US; 2017;31.

[63] Martins-filho ED, Ferraz B, Ferraz EM. Evaluation Of Risk Factors In Superobese Patients Submitted To Conventional Fobi-Capella Surgery. *Arq Gastroenterol.* 2008;45(1):3–10.

[64] Livingston EH, Ko CY. Assessing the Relative Contribution of Individual Risk Factors on Surgical Outcome for Gastric Bypass Surgery : A Baseline Probability Analysis. *J Surg Res*. 2002;105(1):48–52.

[65] Ramanan B, Gupta PK, Gupta H, Fang X, Forse RA. Development and validation of a bariatric surgery mortality risk calculator. *J Am Coll Surg*. Els2012;214(6):892–900.

[66] Caiazzo R, Lassailly G, Leteurtre E, Baud G, Verkindt H, Raverdy V, et al. Roux-en-Y Gastric Bypass Versus Adjustable Gastric Banding to Reduce Nonalcoholic Fatty Liver Disease. *Ann Surg.* 2014;260(5):893–9.

[67] Machado M, Marques-vidal P, Cortez-pinto H. Hepatic histology in obese patients undergoing bariatric surgery. *J Hepatol.* 2006;45(4):600–6.

[68] Losekann A, Weston AC, Carli LA De, Espindola MB, Pioner SR, Coral GP. Nonalcoholic fatty liver disease in severe obese patients, subjected to bariatric surgery. *Arq Gastroenterol*. 2013;50(4): 285–9.

[69] Reha J, Lee S, Hofmann LJ. Prevalence and predictors of nonalcoholic steatohepatitis in obese patients undergoing bariatric surgery: a Department of Defense experience. *Am Surg. Elsevier Inc.*; 2014;80(6):595–9.

[70] Cordeiro L, Campos J, de Paula P, Vilar L, Lopes E, de Arruda P, et al. Nonalcoholic steatohepatitis on preoperative period of gastric

bypass: lack of correlation with degree of obesity. *Arq Bras Cir Dig.* 2013;26(1):39–42.

[71] Wissen J Van, Bakker N, Doodeman HJ. Preoperative Methods to Reduce Liver Volume in Bariatric Surgery : a Systematic Review. *Obes Surg.* 2016;26(2):251–6.

[72] Fris RJ. Preoperative Low Energy Diet Diminishes Liver Size. *Obes Surg.* 2004;14(9):1165–70.

[73] Martínez-Ramos D, Salvador-Sanchis JL, Escrig-Ros J. Pérdida de peso preoperatoria en pacientes candidatos a cirugía bariátrica. Recomendaciones basadas en la evidencia. [Preoperative weight loss in patients candidates for bariatric surgery. Recommendations based on evidence]. *Cir Esp.* 2012;90(3):147–55.

[74] Schwartz ML, Drew RL, Chazin- M. Factors Determining Conversion from Laparoscopic to Open Roux-en-Y Gastric Bypass. *Obes Surg.* 2004;14(9):1193–7.

[75] Schwartz ML, Drew RL, Chazin-Caldie M. Laparoscopic Roux-en-Y Gastric Bypass : Preoperative Determinants of Prolonged Operative Times, Conversion to Open Gastric Bypasses, and Postoperative Complications. *Obes Surg.* 2003;13(5):734–8.

[76] Asad M, Roman K, Johnson S, Afthinos JN, Gibbs KE. Perioperative risk factors for 30-day mortality after bariatric surgery : is functional status important? *Surg Endosc.* 2013;27(5):1772–7.

[77] Consortium LA of BS (LABS), Flum D, Belle S, King W, Wahed A, Berk P, et al. Perioperative Safety in the Longitudinal Assessment of Bariatric Surgery. *N Engl J Med.* 2009;361(5): 445–54.

[78] Turner PL, Saager L, Dalton J, Abd-Elsayed A, Roberman D, Melara P, et al. A nomogram for predicting surgical complications in bariatric surgery patients. *Obes Surg.* 2011;21(5):655–62.

[79] Older P, Smith R, Courtney P, Hone R. Preoperative evaluation of cardiac failure and ischemia in elderly patients by cardiopulmonary exercise testing. *Chest.* 1993;104(3):701–4.

[80] Snowden CP, Prentis JM, Anderson HL, Roberts DR, Randles D, Renton M, et al. Submaximal Cardiopulmonary Exercise Testing Predicts Complications and Hospital Length of Stay in Patients Undergoing Major Elective Surgery. *Ann Surg*. 2010;251(3): 535–41.

[81] Hennis PJ, Meale PM, Hurst RA, Doherty AFO, Otto J, Kuper M, et al. Cardiopulmonary exercise testing predicts postoperative outcome in patients undergoing gastric bypass surgery. *Br J Anaesth.* 2012;109(4):566–71.

[82] McCullough PA, Gallagher MJ, DeJong AT, Sandberg KR, Trivax JE, Alexander D, et al. Cardiorespiratory fitness and short-term complications after bariatric surgery. *Chest.* 2006;130(2):517–25.

[83] Chang S., Stoll C.R.T., Song J., Varela J.E., Eagon C.J., Colditz G.A., The Effectiveness and Risks of Bariatric Surgery An Updated Systematic Review and Meta-analysis, 2003-2012. *JAMA Surg.* 2014;149(3):275–87.

[84] Colles S.L., Dixon J.B., Marks P., Strauss B.J., Brien PEO. Preoperative weight loss with a very-low-energy diet : quantitation of changes in liver and abdominal fat by serial imaging 1–3. *Am J Clin Nutr.* 2006;84(2):304–11.

[85] Edholm D, Kullberg J, Haenni A, Karlsson FA, Ahlström A, Hedberg J, et al. Preoperative 4-week low-calorie diet reduces liver volume and intrahepatic fat, and facilitates laparoscopic gastric bypass in morbidly obese. *Obes Surg.* 2011;21(3):345–50.

[86] Patel N.S., Doycheva I., Peterson M.R., Hooker J., Kisselva T., Schnabl B., et al. Effect of Weight Loss on Magnetic Resonance Imaging Estimation of Liver Fat and Volume in Patients With Nonalcoholic Steatohepatitis. *Clin Gastroenterol Hepatol.* 2015;13(3):561–568.e1.

[87] Tarnoff M, Kaplan LM, Shikora S. An evidenced-based assessment of preoperative weight loss in bariatric surgery. *Obesity Surgery.* 2008;18(9):1059–61.

[88] Benotti PN, Still CD, Wood C, Akmal Y, King H, El Arousy H, et al. Preoperative Weight Loss Before Bariatric Surgery. *Arch Surg.* 2014;144(12):1150–5.

[89] Anderin C, Gustafsson UO, Heijbel N, Thorell A. Weight Loss Before Bariatric Surgery and Postoperative complications. *Ann Surg.* 2015;261(5):909–13.

[90] Gerber P, Anderin C, Thorell A. Weight loss prior to bariatric surgery : An Updated Review of the Literature. *Scand J Surg.* 2014;104(1):33–9.

[91] Nielsen LV, Nielsen MS, Schmidt JB, Sjodin AM. Efficacy of a liquid low calorie formula diet in achieving preoperative target weight loss before bariatric surgery. *J Nutr Sci.* 2016;5:E-22.

[92] Menozzi R, Bondi M, Baldini A, Venneri MG, Velardo A, Del Rio G. Resting metabolic rate, fat-free mass and catecholamine excretion during weight loss in female obese patients. *Br J Nutr.* 2000;84(4):515–20.

[93] Sparti A, Delany JP, De La Bretonne J a., Sander GE, Bray G a. Relationship between resting metabolic rate and the composition of the fat-free mass. *Metabolism.* 1997;46(10):1225–30.

[94] Wu T, Gao X, Chen M, Van Dam RM. Long-term effectiveness of diet-plus-exercise interventions vs. diet-only interventions for weight loss: A meta-analysis: Obesity Management. *Obes Rev.* 2009;10(3):313–23.

[95] Volek JS, Vanheest JL, Forsythe CE. Diet and exercise for weight loss: a review of current issues. *Sport Med.* 2005;35(1):1–9.

[96] Clark JE. Diet, exercise or diet with exercise: comparing the effectiveness of treatment options for weight-loss and changes in fitness for adults (18–65 years old) who are overfat, or obese; systematic review and meta-analysis. *J Diabetes Metab Disord.* 2015;14:31.

[97] Vissers D, Hens W, Taeymans J, Baeyens J-P, Poortmans J, Van Gaal L. The effect of exercise on visceral adipose tissue in overweight adults: a systematic review and meta-analysis. *PLoS One.* 2013;8(2):e56415.

[98] Stiegler P, Cunliffe A. The role of diet and exercise for the maintenance of fat-free mass and resting metabolic rate during weight loss. *Sport Med.* 2006;36(3):239–62.

[99] Mahady SE, George J. Exercise and diet in the management of nonalcoholic fatty liver disease. *Metabolism.* Elsevier B.V.; 2015;65(8):1172–82.

[100] Oliveira CP, Sanches PDL, Abreu-silva EO De, Marcadenti A. Nutrition and Physical Activity in Nonalcoholic Fatty Liver Disease. *J Diabetes Re.* 2016;2016.

[101] Bacchi PE, Moghetti NC, Zanolin ME, Milanese C, Faccioli N, Trombetta M, et al. Metabolic Effects of Aerobic Training and Resistance Training in Type 2 Diabetic Subjects. *Diabetes Care.* 2012;35(4):676–82.

[102] Schwingshackl L, Missbach B, Dias S, König J, Hoffmann G. Impact of different training modalities on glycaemic control and blood lipids in patients with type 2 diabetes: A systematic review and network meta-analysis. *Diabetologia.* 2014;57(9):1789–97.

[103] Schwingshackl L, Dias S, Strasser B, Hoffmann G. Impact of different training modalities on anthropometric and metabolic characteristics in overweight/obese subjects: A systematic review and network meta-analysis. *PLoS One.* 2013;8(12):e82853.

[104] Iftikhar I, Kline C, Youngstedt S. Effects of Exercise Training on Sleep Apnea : A Meta-analysis. *Lung.* 2014;192(1):175–84.

[105] Aiello KD, Caughey WG, Nelluri B, Sharma A, Mookadam F, Mookadam M. Effect of exercise training on sleep apnea: A systematic review and meta-analysis. *Respir Med.* Elsevier Ltd; 2016;116:85–92.

[106] Ruiz-Tovar J, Zubiaga L, Llavero C, Diez M, Arroyo A, Calpena R. Serum cholesterol by morbidly obese patients after laparoscopic sleeve gastrectomy and additional physical activity. *Obes Surg.* 2014;24(3):385–9.

[107] Bond DS, Unick JL, Jakicic JM, Vithiananthan S, Pohl D, Roye GD, et al. Objective Assessment of Time Spent Being Sedentary in Bariatric Surgery Candidates. *Obes Surg.* 2011;21(6):811–4.

[108] Bond D, Jakicic J, Vithiananthan S, Thomas J, Leahey T, Sax H, et al. Objective Quantification of Physical Activity in Bariatric Surgery Candidates and Normal-Weight Controls. *Surg Obes Relat Dis*. 2010;6(1):72–8.

[109] King WC, Belle SH, Eid GM, Dakin GF, Inabnet WB, Mitchell JE, et al. Physical activity levels of patients undergoing bariatric surgery in the Longitudinal Assessment of Bariatric Surgery study. *Surg Obes Relat Dis*. 2008;4(6):721–8.

[110] Freire RH, Borges MC, Alvarez-Leite JI, Toulson Davisson Correia MI. Food quality, physical activity, and nutritional follow-up as determinant of weight regain after Roux-en-Y gastric bypass. *Nutrition*. 2012;28(1):53–8.

[111] Freire RH, Borges MC, Alvarez-Leite JI, Toulson Davisson Correia MI. Food quality, physical activity, and nutritional follow-up as determinant of weight regain after Roux-en-Y gastric bypass. *Nutrition*. 2012;28(1):53–8.

[112] Delgado Floody P, Caamaño Navarrete F, Jerez Mayorga D, Campos Jara C, Ramírez Campillo R, Osorio Poblete A, et al. Efectos de un programa de tratamiento multidisciplinar en obesos mórbidos y obesos con comorbilidades candidatos a cirugía bariátrica [Effects of a multidisciplinary treatment program on morbid and obese obese patients with bariatric surgery comorbidities]. *Nutr Hosp*. 2015;31(5):2011–6.

[113] Delgado Floody P, Jerez Mayorga D, Caamaño Navarrete F, Osorio Poblete A, Thuillier Lepeley N, Alarcón Hormazábal M. Doce semanas de ejercicio físico intervalado con sobrecarga mejora las variables antropométricas de obesos mórbidos y obesos con comorbilidades postulantes a cirugía bariátrica [Twelve weeks of interval physical exercise with overload improves the anthropometric variables of morbid and obese patients with bariatric surgery postoperative comorbidities]. *Nutr Hosp*. 2015;32(5):2007–11.

[114] Delgado Floody P, Cofré Lizama A, Alarcón Hormazábal M, Osorio Poblete A, Caamaño Navarrete F, Jerez Mayorga D.

Evaluación de un programa integral de cuatro meses de duración sobre las condiciones preoperatorias de pacientes obesos candidatos a cirugía bariátrica [Evaluation of a comprehensive four-month program on the preoperative conditions of obese patients who are candidates for bariatric surgery]. *Nutr Hosp*. 2015;32(3):1022–7.

[115] Delgado Floody P, Jerez Mayorga D, Caamano Navarrete F, Concha Diaz M, Ovalle Elgueta H, Osorio Poblete A. [Effectiveness of Comprehensive Treatment on the Preoperative Conditions of Obese Women Candidates for Bariatric Surgery]. *Nutr Hosp*. 2015;32(6):2570–5.

[116] Ortega LS, Juan CS, García AA. Valoración de un programa de ejercicio físico estructurado en pacientes con obesidad mórbida pendientes de cirugía bariátrica [Evaluation of a program of structured physical exercise in patients with morbid obesity awaiting bariatric surgery]. *Nutr Hosp*. 2014;29(1):64–72.

[117] Baillot A, Mampuya WM, Comeau E, Méziat-Burdin A, Langlois MF. Feasibility and impacts of supervised exercise training in subjects with obesity awaiting bariatric surgery: A pilot study. *Obes Surg*. 2013;23(7):882–91.

[118] Marcon ER, Gus I, Neumann CR. Impacto de um programa mínimo de exercícios físicos supervisionados no risco cardiometabólico de pacientes com obesidade mórbida [Impact of a minimum program of supervised physical exercises on the cardiometabolic risk of patients with morbid obesity]. *Arq Bras Endocrinol Metabol*. 2011;55(5):331–8.

[119] Adair JD, Wollner SB, DaCosta ME, Blackburn GL. Progressive Resistance Training for Patients with Class III Obesity. *Obes Weight Manag*. 2010;6(3):115-8.

[120] Marcon ER, Baglioni S, Bittencourt L, Lopes CLN. What Is the Best Treatment before Bariatric Surgery? Exercise, Exercise and Group Therapy, or Conventional Waiting: a Randomized Controlled Trial. *Obes Surg*. 2016;27(3):763–73.

[121] Hickey M, Gavingan K, McCammon M, Tyndall G, Pories W, Israel R, et al. Effects of 7 days of exercise training on insulin action in morbidly obese men. *Clin Exerc Physiol*. 1999;1:24–8.

[122] De Aquino LA, Pereira SE, De Souza Silva J, Sobrinho CJS, Ramalho A. Bariatric surgery: Impact on body composition after Roux-en-Y gastric bypass. *Obes Surg*. 2012;22(2):195–200.

[123] Adamczyk P, Bužga M, Holéczy P, Švagera Z, Šmajstrla V, Zonča P, et al. Bone mineral density and body composition after laparoscopic sleeve gastrectomy in men: A short-term longitudinal study. *Int J Surg*. 2015;23(Pt A):101–7.

[124] Belfiore A, Cataldi M, Minichini L, Aiello ML, Trio R, Rossetti G, et al. Short-Term Changes in Body Composition and Response to Micronutrient Supplementation After Laparoscopic Sleeve Gastrectomy. *Obes Surg*. 2015;25(12):2344–51.

[125] Otto M, Elrefai M, Krammer J, Weiß C, Kienle P, Hasenberg T. Sleeve Gastrectomy and Roux-en-Y Gastric Bypass Lead to Comparable Changes in Body Composition after Adjustment for Initial Body Mass Index. *Obes Surg*. 2015;26(3):479–85.

[126] Calleja-Fernández A, Pintor-de-la-Maza B, Diez-Rodríguez R, Vidal-Casariego A, Urioste-Fondo A, Cano-Rodríguez I, et al. Relationship Between Diet and Body Composition After Biliopancreatic Diversion. *Obes Surg*. 2015;25(11):2093–9.

[127] Carey DG, Pliego GJ, Raymond RL. Body composition and metabolic changes following bariatric surgery: effects on fat mass, lean mass and basal metabolic rate: six months to one-year follow-up. *Obes Surg*. 2006;16(12):1602–8.

[128] Kim MK, Kim W, Kwon HS, Baek KH, Kim EK, Song KH. Effects of bariatric surgery on metabolic and nutritional parameters in severely obese Korean patients with type 2 diabetes: A prospective 2-year follow up. *J Diabetes Investig*. 2014;5(2):221–7.

[129] Busetto L, Tregnaghi A, Marchi F De, Segato G, Foletto M, Sergi G, et al. Liver Volume and Visceral Obesity in Women with Hepatic Steatosis Undergoing Gastric Banding. *Obes Res*. 2002;10(5):408–11.

[130] Cazzo E, Pareja JC, Chaim EA. Nonalcoholic fatty liver disease and bariatric surgery : a comprehensive review. *Sao Paulo Med J.* 2017;135(3):277–95.

[131] Gasteyger C, Suter M, Calmes J. Changes in body composition, metabolic profile and nutritional status 24 months after gastric banding. *Obes Surg*. 2006;16(3):243–50.

[132] Domienik-Karłowicz J, Lisik W, Rymarczyk Z, Dzikowska-Diduch O, Chmura A, Demkow U, et al. The short-term effect of bariatric surgery on non-invasive markers of artery function in patients with metabolic syndrome. *Diabetol Metab Syndr*. 2015;7(1):76.

[133] Lubrano C, Cornoldi A, Pili M, Falcone S, Brandetti F, Fabbrini E, et al. Reduction of risk factors for cardiovascular diseases in morbid-obese patients following biliary-intestinal bypass: 3 years' follow-up. *Int J Obes Relat Metab Disord*. 2004;28(12):1600–6.

[134] Braunwald E, Jensen MD, Fahrbach K. Bariatric Surgery. *Jama.* 2015;292(14):1724.

[135] Kwok CS, Pradhan A, Khan MA, Anderson SG, Keavney BD, Myint PK, et al. Bariatric surgery and its impact on cardiovascular disease and mortality: a systematic review and meta-analysis. *Int J Cardiol*. 2014;173(1):20–8.

[136] Major P, Kowalczuk A, Wysocki M, Osadnik S, Pędziwiatr M, Głuszewska A, et al. Effects of bariatric surgery on cardiovascular risk factors among morbidly obese patients. *Pol Przegl Chir.* 2017;89(1):41–9.

[137] Omotosho P, Mor A, Shantavasinkul PC, Corsino L, Torquati A. Gastric bypass significantly improves quality of life in morbidly obese patients with type 2 diabetes. *Surg Endosc*. 2016;30(7): 2857–64.

[138] Burgmer R, Petersen I, Burgmer M, Zwaan M De, Wolf AM, Herpertz S. Psychological Outcome Two Years after Restrictive *Bariatric Surgery*. 2007;785–91.

[139] Abdeen G, le Roux CW. Mechanism Underlying the Weight Loss and Complications of Roux-en-Y Gastric Bypass. Review. *Obes Surg.* 2016;26(2):410–21.

[140] Stein EM, Silverberg SJ. Bone Loss After Bariatric Surgery: Causes, Consequences and Management. *Lancet Diabetes Endocrinol*. 2014;2(2):165–74.

[141] De Luis DA, Pacheco D, Izaola O, Terroba MC, Cuellar L, Martin T. Clinical results and nutritional consequences of biliopancreatic diversion: Three years of follow-up. *Ann Nutr Metab*. 2009;53(3–4):234–9.

[142] Andreu A, Moizé V, Rodríguez L, Flores L, Vidal J. Protein intake, body composition, and protein status following bariatric surgery. *Obes Surg*. 2010;20(11):1509–15.

[143] Ciangura C, Bouillot J-L, Lloret-Linares C, Poitou C, Veyrie N, Basdevant A, et al. Dynamics of change in total and regional body composition after gastric bypass in obese patients. *Obesity* (Silver Spring). 2010;18(4):760–5.

[144] Carrasco F, Ruz M, Rojas P, Csendes A, Rebolledo A, Codoceo J, et al. Changes in bone mineral density, body composition and adiponectin levels in morbidly obese patients after bariatric surgery. *Obes Surg*. 2009;19(1):41–6.

[145] da Silva FBL, Gomes DL, e Carvalho KMB. Poor diet quality and postoperative time are independent risk factors for weight regain after Roux-en-Y gastric bypass. *Nutrition*. 2016;32:1–4.

[146] Odom J predictors of weight regain after bariatric surgery, Zalesin KC, Washington TL, Miller WW, Hakmeh B, Zaremba DL, et al. Behavioral Predictors ofWeight Regain after Bariatric Surgery. *Obes Surg*. 2010;20(3):349–56.

[147] Faria SL, Kelly E, Faria OP. Energy Expenditure and Weight Regain in Patients Submitted to Roux-en-Y Gastric Bypass. *Obes Surg*. 2009;19(7):856–9.

[148] Felsenreich DM, Langer FB, Kefurt R, Panhofer P, Schermann M, Beckerhinn P, et al. Weight loss, weight regain, and conversions to Roux-en-Y gastric bypass: 10-year results of laparoscopic sleeve gastrectomy. *Surg Obes Relat Dis*. b 2016;12(9):1655–62.

[149] Tamboli RA, Breitman I, Marks-Shulman PA, Jabbour K, Melvin W, Williams B, et al. Early weight regain after gastric bypass does

not affect insulin sensitivity but is associated with elevated ghrelin. *Obesity.* 2014;22(7):1617–22.

[150] Bohdjalian A, Langer FB, Shakeri-Leiden Mühler S, Gfrerer L, Ludvik B, Zacherl J, et al. Sleeve gastrectomy as sole and definitive bariatric procedure: 5-Year results for weight loss and ghrelin. *Obes Surg.* 2010;20(5):535–40.

[151] Herring LY, Stevinson C, Davies MJ, Biddle SJ, Sutton C, Bowrey D, et al. Changes in physical activity behaviour and physical function after bariatric surgery: A systematic review and meta-analysis. *Obes Rev.* 2016;17(3):250–61.

[152] Wouters EJ, Larsen JK, Zijlstra H, Van Ramshorst B, Geenen R. Physical activity after surgery for severe obesity: The role of exercise cognitions. *Obes Surg.* 2011;21(12):1894–9.

[153] Vatier C, Henegar C, Ciangura C, Poitou-Bernert C, Bouillot JL, Basdevant A, et al. Dynamic relations between sedentary behavior, physical activity, and body composition after bariatric surgery. *Obes Surg.* 2012;22(8):1251–6.

[154] Silver HJ, Torquati A, Jensen GL, Richards WO. Weight, dietary and physical activity behaviors two years after gastric bypass. *Obes Surg.* 2006;16(7):859–64.

[155] Colles SL, Dixon JB, O'Brien PE. Hunger Control and Regular Physical Activity Facilitate Weight Loss After Laparoscopic Adjustable Gastric Banding. *Obes Sur.* 2008;18(7):833–40.

[156] Rosenberger PH, Henderson KE, White MA, Masheb RM, Grilo CM. Physical activity in gastric bypass patients: associations with weight loss and psychosocial functioning at 12-month follow-up. *Obes Surg.* 2011;21(10):1564–9.

[157] King W, Hsu J, Belle S, Courcoulas A, Eid G, Flum D, et al. Pre- to Post-operative Changes in Physical Activity: Report from the Longitudinal Assessment of Bariatric Surgery-2. *Surg Obes Relat Dis.* 2012;8(5):522–32.

[158] Jacobi D, Ciangura C, Couet C, Oppert J-M. Physical activity and weight loss following bariatric surgery. *Obes Rev.* 2011;12(5):366–77.

[159] Egberts K, Brown W a, Brennan L, O'Brien PE. Does exercise improve weight loss after bariatric surgery? A systematic review. *Obes Surg*. 2012;22(2):335–41.

[160] Livhits M, Mercado C, Yermilov I, Parikh J a, Dutson E, Mehran A, et al. Exercise following bariatric surgery: systematic review. *Obes Surg*. 2010;20(5):657–65.

[161] Evans RK, Bond DS, Wolfe LG, Meador JG, Herrick JE, Kellum JM, et al. Participation in 150 min/wk of moderate or higher intensity physical activity yields greater weight loss after gastric bypass surgery. *Surg Obes Relat Dis*. 2007;3(5):526–30.

[162] Moya M, Hernández A, Sarabia JM, Sánchez-martos MA, Hernández-davó JL, López-grueso R, et al. Bariatric Surgery, Weight Loss and the Role of Physical Activity : a Systematic Review. *Eur J Hum Mov*. 2014;32:145–60.

[163] Metcalf B, Rabkin R a., Rabkin JM, Metcalf LJ, Lehman-Becker LB. Weight Loss Composition: The Effects of Exercise following Obesity Surgery as Measured by Bioelectrical Impedance Analysis. *Obes Surg*. 2005;15(2):183–6.

[164] Carnero EA, Dubis GS, Hames KC, Jakicic JM, Houmard JA, Coen PM, et al. Randomized Trial Reveals that Physical Activity and Energy Expenditure are Associated with Weight and Body Composition after RYGB. *Obe*s (Silver Spring). 2017;25(7): 1206–16.

[165] Daniels P, Burns RD, Brusseau TA, Hall MS, Adams TD, Eisenman P, et al. Effect of a randomised 12-week resistance training programme on muscular strength, cross- sectional area and muscle quality in women having undergone Roux-en-Y gastric bypass. *J Sports Sci. Routledge*; 2017;1–7.

[166] Campanha-versiani L, Aparecida D, Pereira G, Ribeiro-samora GA, Ramos AV, Fatima M, et al. The Effect of a Muscle Weight-Bearing and Aerobic Exercise Program on the Body Composition, Muscular Strength, Biochemical Markers, and Bone Mass of Obese Patients Who Have Undergone Gastric Bypass Surgery. *Obes Surg*. 2017;27(8):2129–37.

[167] Muschitz C, Kocijan R, Haschka J, Zendeli A, Pirker T, Geiger C, et al. The Impact of Vitamin D, Calcium, Protein Supplementation, and Physical Exercise on Bone Metabolism after Bariatric Surgery: The BABS Study. *J Bone Miner Res*. 2016;31(3):672–82.

[168] Hassannejad A, Khalaj A, Mansournia MA, Tabesh MR, Alizadeh Z. The Effect of Aerobic or Aerobic-Strength Exercise on Body Composition and Functional Capacity in Patients with BMI ≥ 35 after Bariatric Surgery : a Randomized Control. Obes Surg. *Obesity Surgery*; 2017;27(11):2792–801.

[169] Castello V, Simões RP, Bassi D, Catai AM, Arena R, Borghi-Silva A. Impact of aerobic exercise training on heart rate variability and functional capacity in obese women after gastric bypass surgery. *Obes Surg*. 2011;21(11):1739–49.

[170] Stegen S, Derave W, Calders P, Van Laethem C, Pattyn P. Physical fitness in morbidly obese patients: effect of gastric bypass surgery and exercise training. *Obes Surg*. 2011;21(1):61–70.

[171] Faria SL, Faria OP, Buffington C, De Almeida Cardeal M, Rodrigues De Gouvêa H. Energy expenditure before and after Roux-en-Y gastric bypass. *Obes Surg*. 2012;22(9):1450–5.

[172] Sumithran P, Proietto J. The defence of body weight: a physiological basis for weight regain after weight loss. *Clin Sci* (Lond). 2013;124(4):231–41.

[173] Browning MG, Franco RL, Cyrus JC, Celi F, Evans RK. Changes in Resting Energy Expenditure in Relation to Body Weight and Composition Following Gastric Restriction : A Systematic Review. *Obes Surg*. 2016;26(7):1607–15.

[174] Wiklund M, Olsén MF, Olbers T, Cider Å. Physical fitness and physical activity in Swedish women before and one year after roux-en-y gastric bypass surgery. *Open Obes J*. 2015;6(1):38–43.

[175] Lund MT, Hansen M, Wimmelmann CL, Taudorf LR, Helge JW, Mortensen EL, et al. Increased post-operative cardiopulmonary fitness in gastric bypass patients is explained by weight loss. *Scand J Med Sci Sports*. 2015;n/a-n/a. A.

[176] Wilms B, Ernst B, Thurnheer M, Weisser B, Schultes B. Differential changes in exercise performance after massive weight loss induced by bariatric surgery. *Obes Surg*. 2013;23(3):365–71.

[177] Huck CJ. Effects of Supervised Resistance Training on Fitness And Functional Strength in Patients Succeeding Bariatric Surgery. *J strength Cond Res*. 2015;29(3):589–95.

[178] Shah M, Snell PG, Rao S, Adams-Huet B, Quittner C, Livingston EH, et al. High-volume exercise program in obese bariatric surgery patients: a randomized, controlled trial. *Obesity* (Silver Spring). 2011;19(9):1826–34.

[179] Coen PM, Tanner CJ, Helbling NL, Dubis GS, Hames KC, Xie H, et al. Clinical trial demonstrates exercise following bariatric surgery improves insulin sensitivity. *J Clin Invest*. 2015;125(1):248–57.

[180] Wei M, Kampert JB, Barlow CE, Nichaman MZ, Gibbons LW, Paffenbarger RS, et al. Relationship between low cardiorespiratory fitness and mortality in normal-weight, overweight, and obese men. *JAMA*. 1999;282(16):1547–53.

[181] DeFina LF, Haskell WL, Willis BL, Barlow CE, Finley CE, Levine BD, et al. Physical Activity Versus Cardiorespiratory Fitness: Two (Partly) Distinct Components of Cardiovascular Health? *Prog Cardiovasc Dis*. 2015;57(4):324–9.

[182] Gilbertson NM, Paisley AS, Kranz S, Weltman A, Kirby JL, Hallowell PT, et al. Bariatric Surgery Resistance: Using Preoperative Lifestyle Medicine and/or Pharmacology for Metabolic Responsiveness. *Obes Surg. Obesity Surgery*; 2017;27(12):3281–91.

[183] Shada AL, Hallowell PT, Schirmer BD, Smith PW. Aerobic exercise is associated with improved weight loss after laparoscopic adjustable gastric banding. *Obes Surg*. 2013;23(5):608–12.

[184] Wefers JF, Woodlief TL, Carnero EA, Helbling NL, Anthony SJ, Dubis GS, et al. Relationship among physical activity, sedentary behaviors, and cardiometabolic risk factors during gastric bypass surgery-induced weight loss. *Surg Obes Relat Dis Off J Am Soc Bariatr Surg*. 2016;1–10.

[185] Woodlief TL, Carnero EA, Standley RA, Distefano G, Anthony SJ, Dubis GS, et al. Dose Response of Exercise Training Following Roux-en-Y Gastric Bypass Surgery : A Randomized Trial. *Obes* (Silver Spring). 2015;23(12):2454–61.

[186] Schauer DP, Arterburn DE, Livingston EH, Coleman KJ, Ph D, Sidney S, et al. Impact of bariatric surgery on life expectancy in severely obese patients with diabetes: A Decision analysis. *Ann Surg.* 2016;261(5):914–9.

[187] Magro DO, Geloneze B, Delfini R, Pareja BC, Callejas F, Pareja JC. Long-term weight regain after gastric bypass: A 5-year prospective study. *Obes Surg*. 2008;18(6):648–51.

[188] Gomes DL, de Almeida Oliveira D, Dutra ES, Pizato N, de Carvalho KMB. Resting Energy Expenditure and Body Composition of Women with Weight Regain 24 Months After Bariatric Surgery. *Obes Surg*. 2015.

[189] Himpens J, Dobbeleir J, Peeters G. Long-term results of laparoscopic sleeve gastrectomy for obesity. *Ann Surg*. 2010;252(2):319–24.

[190] Sarela AI, Dexter SPL, O'Kane M, Menon A, McMahon MJ. Long-term follow-up after laparoscopic sleeve gastrectomy: 8-9-year results. *Surg Obes Relat Dis*. 2012;8(6):679–84.

[191] Shah M, Simha V, Garg A. Review: long-term impact of bariatric surgery on body weight, comorbidities, and nutritional status. *J Clin Endocrinol Metab* 2006;91(11):4223–31.

[192] Sjöström L, Lindroos A, Peltonen M, Torgerson J, Bouchard C, Carlsson B, et al. Lifestyle, Diabetes, and Cardiovascular Risk Factors 10 Years after Bariatric Surgery. *N Engl J Med.* 2004;351(26):2683–93.

[193] Golomb I, Ben David M, Glass A, Kolitz T, Keidar A. Long-term Metabolic Effects of Laparoscopic Sleeve Gastrectomy. *JAMA Surg.* 2015;150(11):1051–7.

[194] Arterburn DE, Bogart A, Sherwood NE, Sidney S, Coleman KJ, Haneuse S, et al. A multisite study of long-term remission and

relapse of type 2 diabetes mellitus following gastric bypass. *Obes Surg.* 2013;23(1):93–102.

[195] Brethauer SA, Aminian A, Romero-Talamás H, Batayyah E, Mackey J, Kennedy L, et al. Can diabetes be surgically cured? Long-term metabolic effects of bariatric surgery in obese patients with type 2 diabetes mellitus. *Ann Surg.* 2013;258(4):628-36-7.

[196] Dogan K, Betzel B, Homan J, Aarts EO, Ploeger N, de Boer H, et al. Long-Term Effects of Laparoscopic Roux-en-Y Gastric Bypass on Diabetes Mellitus, Hypertension and Dyslipidaemia in Morbidly Obese Patients. *Obes Surg.* 2014;24(11):1835–42.

[197] Jimenez A, Casamitjana R, Flores L, Viaplana J, Corcelles R, Lacy A, et al. Long-Term Effects of Sleeve Gastrectomy and Roux-en-Y Gastric Bypass Surgery on Type 2 Diabetes Mellitus in Morbidly Obese Subjects. *Ann Surg.* 2012;256(6):1023–9. A

[198] Benaiges D, Sagué M, Roux JAF, Pedro-botet J, Ramón JM, Chillarón JJ, et al. Predictors of Hypertension Remission and Recurrence After Bariatric Surgery. *Am J Hypertens.* 2016;29(5):653–9.

[199] King WC, Chen J, Bond DS, Belle SH, Courcoulas AP, Patterson EJ, et al. Objective Assessment of Changes in Physical Activity and Sedentary Behavior : Pre- Through 3 Years Post-Bariatric Surgery. *Obes* (Silver Spring). 2015;23(6):1143–50.

[200] Herman KM, Carver TE, Christou N V, Andersen RE. Keeping the weight off: Physical activity, sitting time, and weight loss maintenance in bariatric surgery patients 2 to 16 years postsurgery. *Obes Surg.* 2014;24(7):1064–72.

[201] Herman KM, Carver TE, Christou N V., Andersen RE. Keeping the weight off: Physical activity, sitting time, and weight loss maintenance in bariatric surgery patients 2 to 16 years postsurgery. *Obes Surg.* 2014;24:1064–72.

[202] Papalazarou A, Yannakoulia M, Kavouras S a, Komesidou V, Dimitriadis G, Papakonstantinou A, et al. Lifestyle intervention favorably affects weight loss and maintenance following obesity surgery. *Obesity (*Silver Spring). 2010;18(7):1348–53.

[203] Kalarchian MA, Marcus MD, Courcoulas AP, Cheng Y, Levine MD, Josbeno D. Optimizing long-term weight control after bariatric surgery: a pilot study. *Surg Obes Relat Dis*. Elsevier Inc.; 2012;8(6):710–5.

[204] Herring LY, Stevinson C, Carter P, Biddle SJH, Bowrey D, Sutton C, et al. The effects of supervised exercise training 12 – 24 months after bariatric surgery on physical function and body composition: a randomised controlled trial. *Int J Obes*. Nature Publishing Group; 2017;41(6):909–16.

[205] Hainer V, Toplak H, Mitrakou A. Treatment modalities of obesity: what fits whom? *Diabetes Care*. 2008;31(Suppl 2):S269-277.

[206] Donnelly JE, Blair SN, Jakicic JM, Manore MM, Rankin JW, Smith BK. Appropriate Physical Activity Intervention Strategies for Weight Loss and Prevention of Weight Regain for Adults. *Medicine and Science in Sports and Exercise*. 2009. p. 459–71.

[207] Jakicic JM, Clark K, Coleman E, Donnelly JE, Foreyt J, Melanson E, et al. American College of Sports Medicine position stand. Appropriate intervention strategies for weight loss and prevention of weight regain for adults. *Med Sci Sports Exerc*. 2001;33(12): 2145–56.

[208] Tresierras M a, Balady GJ. Resistance training in the treatment of diabetes and obesity: mechanisms and outcomes. *J Cardiopulm Rehabil Prev*. 2008;29:67–75.

[209] Strasser B, Schobersberger W. Evidence for resistance training as a treatment therapy in obesity. *J Obes*. 2011;482564.

[210] Schwingshackl L, Dias S, Strasser B, Hoffmann G. Impact of different training modalities on anthropometric and metabolic characteristics in overweight/obese subjects: a systematic review and network meta-analysis. *PLoS One*. 2013;8(12):e82853.

[211] Ho SS, Dhaliwal SS, Hills AP, Pal S. The effect of 12 weeks of aerobic, resistance or combination exercise training on cardiovascular risk factors in the overweight and obese in a randomized trial. *BMC Public Health*. 2012;12:704.

[212] Willis LH, Slentz C a, Bateman L a, Shields a T, Piner LW, Bales CW, et al. Effects of aerobic and/or resistance training on body mass and fat mass in overweight or obese adults. *J Appl Physiol.* 2012;113(12):1831–7.

[213] Sanal E, Ardic F, Kirac S. Effects of aerobic or combined aerobic resistance exercise on body composition in overweight and obese adults: Gender differences. A randomized intervention study. *Eur J Phys Rehabil Med.* 2013;49(1):1–11.

[214] Park S-K, Park J-H, Kwon Y-C, Kim H-S, Yoon M-S, Park H-T. The effect of combined aerobic and resistance exercise training on abdominal fat in obese middle-aged women. *J Physiol Anthropol Appl Human Sci.* 2003;22(3):129–35.

[215] Dâmaso AR, Campos RMDS, Caranti DA, de Piano A, Fisberg M, Foschini D, et al. Aerobic plus resistance training was more effective in improving the visceral adiposity, metabolic profile and inflammatory markers than aerobic training in obese adolescents. *J Sports Sci.* 2014;32:1–11.

[216] Buchheit M, Laursen PB. High-intensity interval training, solutions to the programming puzzle: Part I: cardiopulmonary emphasis. *Sports Med.* 2013;43(5):313–38.

[217] Laforgia J, Withers RT, Gore CJ. Effects of exercise intensity and duration on the excess post-exercise oxygen consumption. *J Sports Sci.* 2006;24(12):1247–64.

[218] Børsheim E, Bahr R. Effect of exercise intensity, duration and mode on post-exercise oxygen consumption. *Sport Med.* 2003; 33(14):1037–60.

[219] Perry CGR, Heigenhauser GJF, Bonen A, Spriet LL. High-intensity aerobic interval training increases fat and carbohydrate metabolic capacities in human skeletal muscle. *Appl Physiol Nutr Metab.* 2008;33(6):1112–23.

[220] Whyte LJ, Ferguson C, Wilson J, Scott R a., Gill JMR. Effects of single bout of very high-intensity exercise on metabolic health biomarkers in overweight/obese sedentary men. *Metabolism.* 2013;62(2):212–9.

[221] Wewege M, van den Berg R, Ward RE, Keech A. The effects of high-intensity interval training vs. moderate-intensity continuous training on body composition in overweight and obese adults: a systematic review and meta-analysis. *Obes Rev*. 2017;18(6):635-646.

[222] Racil G, Ben Ounis O, Hammouda O, Kallel A, Zouhal H, Chamari K, et al. Effects of high vs. moderate exercise intensity during interval training on lipids and adiponectin levels in obese young females. *Eur J Appl Physiol*. 2013;113(10):2531–40.

[223] Alvarez L, Ramírez-Campillo R, Flores O, Henríquez-Olguín C, Campos J, Carrasco V, et al. Metabolic response to high intensity exercise training in sedentary hyper- glycemic and hypercholesterolemic women. *Rev Med Chil*. 2013;141(10):1293–9.

[224] Paoli A, Pacelli QF, Moro T, Marcolin G, Neri M, Battaglia G, et al. Effects of high-intensity circuit training, low-intensity circuit training and endurance training on blood pressure and lipoproteins in middle-aged overweight men. *Lipids Health Dis*. 2013;12(3):131.

[225] Jelleyman C, Yates T, O'Donovan G, Gray LJ, King JA, Khunti K, et al. The effects of high-intensity interval training on glucose regulation and insulin resistance: A meta-analysis. *Obes Rev*. 2015;16(11):942–61.

[226] Batacan RB, Duncan MJ, Dalbo VJ, Tucker PS, Fenning AS. Effects of high-intensity interval training on cardiometabolic health: a systematic review and meta-analysis of intervention studies. *Br J Sports Med*. 2016;51(6):494–503.

[227] Milanović Z, Sporiš G, Weston M. Effectiveness of High-Intensity Interval Training (HIT) and Continuous Endurance Training for VO2max Improvements: A Systematic Review and Meta-Analysis of Controlled Trials. *Sport Med*. 2015;45(10):1469–81.

[228] Kessler HS, Sisson SB, Short KR. The potential for high-intensity interval training to reduce cardiometabolic disease risk. *Sport Med*. 2012;42(6):489–509.

[229] Kelley DE. Skeletal muscle fat oxidation: timing and flexibility are everything. *J Clin Invest*. 2005;115(7):1699–702.

[230] Davidson LE, Hudson R, Kilpatrick K, Kuk JL, McMillan K, Janiszewski PM, Lee S, Lam M, Ross R. Effects of exercise modality on insulin resistance and functional limitation in older adults: a randomized controlled trial. *Arch Intern Med*. 2009;26;169(2):122-31.

[231] Snowling NJ, Hopkins WG. Effects of different modes of exercise training on glucose control and risk factors for complications in type 2 diabetic patients: a meta-analysis. *Diabetes Care*. 2006; 29(11):2518- 2527.

In: A Closer Look at Cardiovascular … ISBN: 978-1-53613-939-6
Editor: Faris van Kilsdonk

Chapter 2

ENDOTHELIAL DYSFUNCTION: MORE THAN A NEW CARDIOVASCULAR RISK FACTOR

Cotugno Annunziata, Fabbricatore Davide, Vizzardi Enrico, Gavazzoni Mara, Bonadei Ivano, Sciatti Edoardo, Valentini Francesca, Scodro Marta, Castiello Assunta, Perego Carlotta, Raddino Riccardo and Metra Marco

Division of Cardiology, Department of Medical and Surgical Specialties, Radiological Sciences, and Public Health, University and Civil Hospital of Brescia, Brescia, Italy

ABSTRACT

Endothelial dysfunction is a well-described precursor to the development of clinically overt coronary and peripheral artery disease and is present early in the course of the disease. It reflects not only the global atherosclerotic status, but also the degree of rigidity of the whole artery system, thus representing an independent predictor of future CV events and all-cause mortality. The measurement of endothelial function could therefore represent an additional prognostic marker of cardiovascular risk.

The current gold standard methods to evaluate the endothelial function are intracoronary or intra-brachial infusions of vasoactive agents that enhance the release of endothelial nitric oxide (such as acetylcholine and bradykinin) and offer direct quantification of vascular response to NO. However these tests are invasive, expensive and not easily reliable.

Hence it appears clear the urge to find methods that could evaluate the endothelial function in an easier and not invasive way. In this sense various techniques have been tested in the recent past, but only two of them have shown a similar and strong correlation with cardiovascular risk compared to the invasive methods.

The more widely used is Brachial artery flow-mediated dilatation (FMD) which is based on ultrasound measures of flow-mediated changes in arterial diameter in superficial arteries (for example the brachial, radial or femoral vessels). This changes are caused by shear-stress induced generation of endothelial derived vasoactive mediators, especially represented by NO.

A more recent method is Peripheral arterial tonometry (PAT) that uses fingertip plethysmography to measure pulse volume amplitude: its changes in response to hyperemia have been shown to be nitric oxide (NO)-dependent. This suggests that PAT is a measure of endothelial function.

Despite these methods give an indirect estimate of endothelial function, the studies that evaluated FMD and PAT showed that they are independent CV risk factors and predictors of CV events and all-cause mortality. This is even more evident in the population with previously assessed CVD or with other CV risk factors.

Further research to evaluate the prognostic utility of both these methods (especially for the more recent PAT) is necessary to compare them with invasive endothelial function test in clinical practice.

1. INTRODUCTION

Endothelial dysfunction is well known to be precursor of coronary and peripheral artery disease, predictor of future cardiovascular (CV) events and all-cause mortality. Indeed, measurement of endothelial function could represent an additional prognostic marker of cardiovascular risk.

The current gold standard methods to evaluate the endothelial function are intracoronary or intra-brachial infusions of vasoactive agents that cause releasing of endothelial nitric oxide (NO) (such as acetylcholine and bradykinin), allowing direct quantification of vascular response to NO. However these tests are invasive, expensive and not easily reliable.

Noninvasive tests for the assessment of coronary endothelial function include Doppler echography, phase-contrast magnetic resonance imaging, flow mediated dilation (FMD) and Peripheral Artery Tonometry (PAT). The last two methods (which are "indirect" methods) represent the most widely used noninvasive techniques for the evaluation of endothelial function.

Several evidence does exist to support the role of these methods in predicting cardiovascular events, both in primary and secondary prevention setting [1].

The research of new CV risk factors beyond the "traditional" ones became necessary because the latter failed to demonstrate sufficient sensitivity and specificity in predicting events in individual patients and cannot provide a clear clinical route for identification or treatment of near-future victims of acute coronary syndrome or sudden death [2-4].

2. Endothelial Function: Physiopathology

Up to 40 years ago, endothelium was considered only a "passive" monolayer between the blood torrent and the interstitial space of the organs, playing a role in blood coagulation processes.

During the last years, it has been shown that the vascular endothelium is more than a simple "coating or monolayer" and nowadays it's considered the most important autocrine and paracrine organ. It's not a surprise by taking in consideration its weight (around 2 Kg) and its width of around 400 m^2 and the fact that it is made up of more than a billion nucleate cells.

It produces and responds to several vasoactive molecules that influence the motion of vessels. Therefore, it plays a direct role in the balance of tissue oxygen supply and metabolic demand by regulation of vessel tone and diameter, and it is involved in the remodeling of vascular structure and long-term organ perfusion [5].

The normal endothelial function depends on both the continuity of the cellular layer and its functional integrity.

The studies of Furchgott and Zawadzki first demonstrated the importance of the endothelium integrity in ensuring the right functioning to the whole vascular system. They identified an endothelium-derived relaxing factor (EDRF) which mediated the endothelium dependent vasodilation [6].

After some years, nitric oxide (NO) was recognized to be this endothelium-derived relaxing factor [7].

This discovery was so important to allow Furchgott, Ignarro and Murad to win the Nobel Prize for physiology and medicine in 1998.

NO is a gaseous molecule, generated from L-arginine by the action of endothelial NO synthase (eNOS) in the presence of cofactors like Dihydronicotinamide-adenine dinucleotide phosphate (NADPH), Flavin Mono Nucleotide (FMN), Flavin adenine dinucleotide (FAD) and tetrahydrobiopterin (H4B).

The chemical structure of NO presents an unpaired electron that gives a great deal of reactivity to the molecule.

Due to its instability, this gas has a short half-life (taking about 5 seconds) but is able to diffuse to the vascular smooth muscle cells and activate soluble guanylate cyclase, which leads to generation of cyclic guanosine monophosphate (cGMP) -mediated vasodilatation.

Several substances contributing to the physiological activity of the e-NOS, for example: acetylcholine, bradykinin, adenosine, substance P, vascular endothelial growth factor (in response to hypoxia), and serotonin (released during platelet aggregation).

The extent of vasodilatation induced by some of these substances, as described later in the lecture, represents a measure of endothelial function.

Beyond these chemical factors, there are also other mechanical elements that play a role in this activation, such as the shear stress, which acts with a mechanism independent from a binding to a receptor, and still not fully clarified [8].

The endothelium also mediates hyperpolarization of vascular smooth muscle cells via a NO-independent pathway, which increases potassium conductance and subsequent propagation of depolarization of vascular smooth muscle cells.

On the other hand the endothelium can cause vasoconstriction by producing endothelin and vasoconstrictor prostanoids, as well as converting angiotensin I to angiotensin II at its surface.

These vasoconstrictor agents act locally on the arterial wall, but they have also some systemic effects and have a role in the regulation structure and remodeling of arterial and the heart [9-12].

In vascular physiology, the continuous release of NO helps to keep the vascular wall in a quiescent state by inhibition of inflammation, cellular proliferation, and thrombosis.

This is in part achieved by s-nitrosylation of cysteine residues in a wide range of proteins, which reduces their biological activity. The target proteins include the transcription factor NFκB, cell cycle–controlling proteins, and proteins involved in generation of tissue factor [13].

All of these mechanisms can be altered in a state of endothelial dysfunction. The imbalance between vaso-dilating and constrictor substances leads to an inappropriate endothelium-dependent vasodilation, which is the functional characteristic of endothelial dysfunction.

In addition to impaired endothelium-dependent vasodilation, endothelial dysfunction also involves a specific state of endothelial activation, which is characterized by a pro-inflammatory, proliferative, and pro-coagulant state that promotes all stages of atherogenesis [14].

The endothelium also acts on the platelet activity, releasing continuously substances like prostacyclin and NO that inhibit the adhesion and aggregation of platelets to the vessel wall (by the increase of cAMP and cGMP intra-platelet concentration and calcium release) [15].

Thus endothelial dysfunction also leads to inappropriate platelets aggregation.

Furthermore, the integrity of the endothelium monolayer is the most important inhibitor of intimal hyperplasia, because it represents a physical barrier to the passage of leukocytes and platelets [16].

When it is removed (artificially in the laboratories) or damaged (*in vivo*), it allows cells passage inducing vascular smooth muscle proliferation [17].

Considering the relationship between all these processes (endothelial dysfunction) and atherosclerosis, they could directly reflect the propensity to develop atherosclerotic disease.

3. Measurement of Endothelial Function

The current gold standard methods to evaluate the endothelial function are intracoronary or intra-brachial infusions of vasoactive agents that enhance the release of endothelial nitric oxide (such as acetylcholine and bradykinin) and offer direct quantification of vascular response to NO. However these tests are invasive, expensive and not easily reliable.

Hence it appears clear the urge to find methods that could evaluate the endothelial function in an easier and not invasive way. In this sense various techniques have been tested in the recent past, but only two of them have shown a similar and strong correlation with cardiovascular risk compared to the invasive methods.

The more widely used is Brachial artery flow-mediated dilatation (FMD), which is based on ultrasound measures of flow-mediated changes in arterial diameter in superficial arteries (for example the brachial, radial or femoral vessels). This changes are caused by shear-stress induced generation of endothelial derived vasoactive mediators, especially represented by NO.

A more recent method is Peripheral Arterial Tonometry (PAT) that uses fingertip plethysmography to measure pulse volume amplitude: its changes in response to hyperemia have been shown to be nitric oxide (NO)-dependent. This suggests that PAT is a measure of endothelial function.

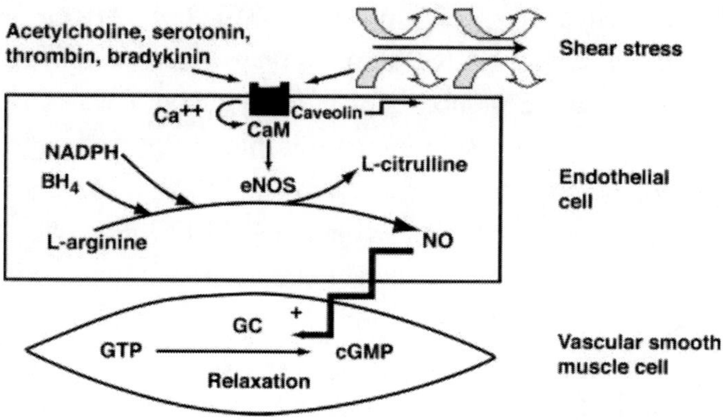

Figure 1. From Jean Davignon, Peter Ganz; Role of Endothelial Dysfunction in atherosclerosis. Circulation 2004;109:III-27-III-32.

Another non-invasive method for the assessment of endothelial function is represented by Cardiovascular Magnetic Resonance (CMR).

In particular, coronary endothelial function can be quantified non-invasively with ECG-triggered spiral cine MRI combined with isometric handgrip exercise (IHE).

The standard approach involves synchronized acquisition of the ECG; however, recently, it has been tested new methods without ECG triggered acquisitions, with good results [18-19].

Different studies showed that measurements of endothelial function obtained with MRI correlate to coronary dysfunction in different situations, such as smoking, diabetes or aging [20-23].

However, this methodical cannot be routinely used because of its prolonged procedural times and its high costs so it won't be further deepened in this chapter.

3.1. Invasive Methods

First clinical studies to test endothelial function were performed in the coronary circulation using invasive assessment, and angiography still represents the gold standard for measuring endothelial function [24].

Vasoactive substances with a vasodilatory effect, especially acetylcholine, are administrated into coronary arteries through cardiac catheterization. These substances activate endothelial cells to release NO, thus producing vasodilation and increase in blood flow. Changes in artery diameter and blood flow are measured by quantitative angiography and a Doppler system. In patients with endothelial dysfunction, we observe an impaired response or even a vasoconstriction without increase in coronary blood flow, caused by direct activation of muscarinic receptors on vascular smooth muscle cells [25].

In patients undergoing coronary catheterization for ischemic heart disease, with this technique, it was demonstrated the presence of endothelial dysfunction in coronary atherosclerosis and its prognostic significance in predicting disease progression and cardiovascular events [25, 26].

Since then, the attention was focused on microvascular function and it was demonstrated that, also without evidence of coronary plaques, endothelial dysfunction at this level, assessed with coronary catheterization and Acetylcholine (ACh) administration, is a predictor of future cardiovascular events and coronary artery disease progression [27-29].

Of course, being an invasive method, it cannot be used in daily practice and, also in the field of clinical trials, it is not normally conducted unless there is another clinical reason for intra-coronary catheterization. Hence the need to test and validate non-invasive techniques which could be less expensive, easily applied and reproducible, and give overlapping results with respect to angiography.

3.2. Non-Invasive Methods

3.2.1. Flow-mediated Dilation (FMD)

As previously stated, FMD evaluated with Brachial Artery Ultrasound Imaging represents one of the most widely used non-invasive technique to measure endothelial function. It estimates the ability of the arteries to respond to reactive hyperemia with endothelial release of vasoactive substance [30-33].

As recent guidelines explain [34, 35, 36], this technique requires extensive training and standardization to obtain homogeneous data from different operators. It is necessary to carefully prepare the subject, to establish site selection and sphygmomanometer probe position, cuff occlusion time and correct characterization of the FMD response, so the reproducibility of FMD can be considerably improved [37, 38, 34, 39].

Endothelial dysfunction is reflected in an impaired FMD response, which is mainly NO-dependent [39, 36, 30, 31, 32, 33].

The reference technique is that described by Celermajer et al. [40]: the brachial artery diameter proximal to the antecubital fossa is measured at rest and during reactive hyperemia. The latter is obtained by rapid release of a pneumatic pressure cuff placed around the forearm and inflated to supra-systolic pressure for 5 minutes. The FMD, which is endothelium dependent, is expressed as the change in the final diastolic diameter of the brachial artery compared with the baseline value. This measurement should be taken at the end of diastole, so it is necessary to have simultaneous monitoring of the electrocardiogram. An absent or reduced vasodilation suggests decreased release of endogenous vasoactive substances in response to increase shear stress (i.e., endothelial dysfunction).

The standard technique involves determination of the diameter at a fixed time point, usually 60 seconds after cuff deflation. However, studies demonstrated that this method underestimated the maximal FMD response [41]. There are evidences that the use of continuous diameter measurements are more effective and reliable in providing information about endothelial function both in healthy subjects and in patients with cardiovascular disease [42-43].

It is also important to notice that different cuff positions influence FMD response: the more proximal the occlusion, the greater the vasodilatory response [44]. Also the baseline diameter is a variable to consider: arteries with larger baseline diameter will face less dilation than smaller ones.

Of course measurements acquired with FMD significantly depends on physiological and pathophysiological factors: for example hormones, especially for women and also for the same woman in different phases of menstrual cycle, and other systemic conditions that cause increased sympathetic tone, such as hypertension and renal failure [45].

It has been widely demonstrated that FMD provides independent prognostic information about risk of cardiovascular events both in patients with established cardiovascular diseases and in asymptomatic subjects. The fundamental aspect is that FMD has not only the same predictive value of traditional risk factors, but may also provide additional prognostic individual information about cardiovascular risk [46, 47].

Moreover, several trials have not shown an evident correlation between brachial FMD and the carotid intima media thickness (IMT); however, it seems to correlate with IMT progression over years in a population free of cardiovascular and atherosclerotic disease, better than other validated and more used risk index (i.e., Framingham Risk Score). [48, 49].

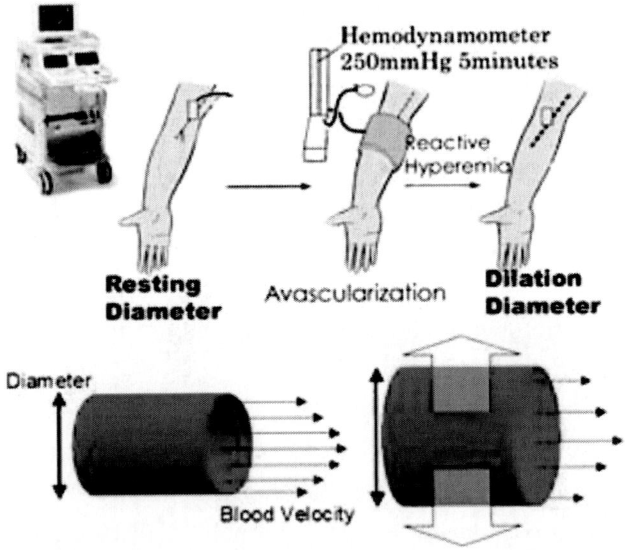

Figure 2. Flow-mediated dilatation from Study on automatic FMD, Dept. Of Environmental Studies, University of Tokyo.

Thus, it could be useful, for example, to perform a noninvasive test of endothelial function in selected healthy patients (i.e., patients with familiarity with CAD), taking basal measurements and repeating them after a defined period to detect a subclinical dysfunction

3.2.2. Low Flow Mediated Constriction (LFMC)

Low Flow mediated constriction (LFMC) measures resting endothelial activity. It is calculated as the decrease in arterial diameter in the last 30 seconds of cuff occlusion (after 4,5 minutes) compared with baseline diameter [50]. It expresses the response of conduit arteries to a decrease in blood flow and shear stress [51].

It has been demonstrated that there is not correlation between FMD and LFMC (28), thus indicating that different substances are responsible for the response to increased or reduced shear stress. Indeed, while FMD reflects mainly synthesis and release of NO, LFMC is the result of the production of different vasoactive substances, such as vasodilators (i.e., prostaglandins) and vasoconstrictors (i.e., endothelin-1). [50, 52].

The information provided by LFMC are complementary with respect to FMD, representing another possible method to predict cardiovascular risk non-invasively, in addiction to traditional risk factors.

3.2.3. Peripheral Arterial Tonometry (PAT)

Peripheral arterial tonometry (PAT) is a more recent noninvasive method to evaluate endothelial function. It uses fingertip plethysmography to measure pulse volume amplitude and its changes in response to reactive hyperemia. Since it has been demonstrated that this parameter is dependent on the nitric oxide action, it's possible to assess that PAT represents a method to measure endothelial function, in particular at microvascular level, with an easy to perform and operator independent technique.

On the other hand PAT seems to be influenced by non-endothelial factors and less dependent on NO release [24].

It involves a finger-mounted probe tonometer plethysmograph that detect the volume changes in the vessels of the index finger during each pulsation. The index is the most appropriated finger because of the presence of adequate vascularization and the absence of major muscle masses. The probes apply a constant pressure (70 mmHg) across the finger. Two probes are used, one for each hand; at the same time a blood pressure cuff is inflated over systolic pressure in one arm (tested arm). The contemporary assessment of PAT signal from both texted and control arm allows internal control, to reduce influence of factors as: external stressors, sympathetic activation, pharmacological modulation.

PAT signal is recorded for 5 minutes at baseline, 5 minutes during pressure-cuff inflating and 5 minutes after deflating of cuff. Reactive hyperemia is obtained releasing the cuff in the test arm and the signal is recorded for 5 minutes. Normally, during the reactive hyperemia, the blood flow increases. Also the pulse amplitude rises in healthy individuals, whereas a low response is observed in subjects with endothelial dysfunction. A software elaborates the signals during all phases and the final output is the reactive hyperemia index (RHI), which is the ratio of average amplitude during reactive hyperemia and the pre-occlusion baseline period one, multiplied by the baseline correction factor ($0.2276 \times \ln$ (mean occluded baseline amplitude) $- 0.2$) [53].

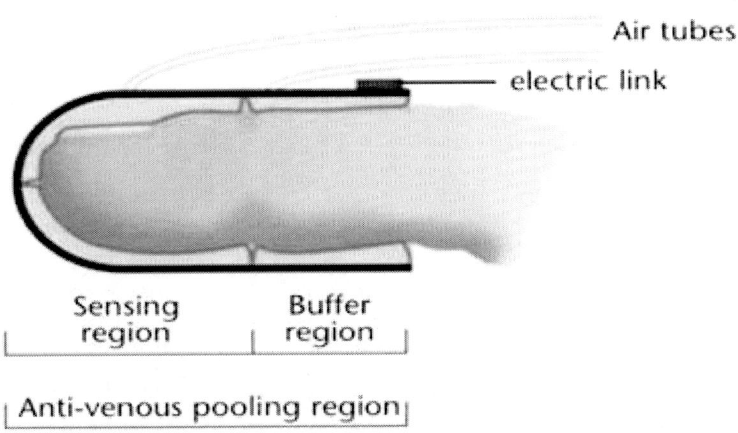

Figure 3. Probe for endoPAT evaluation.

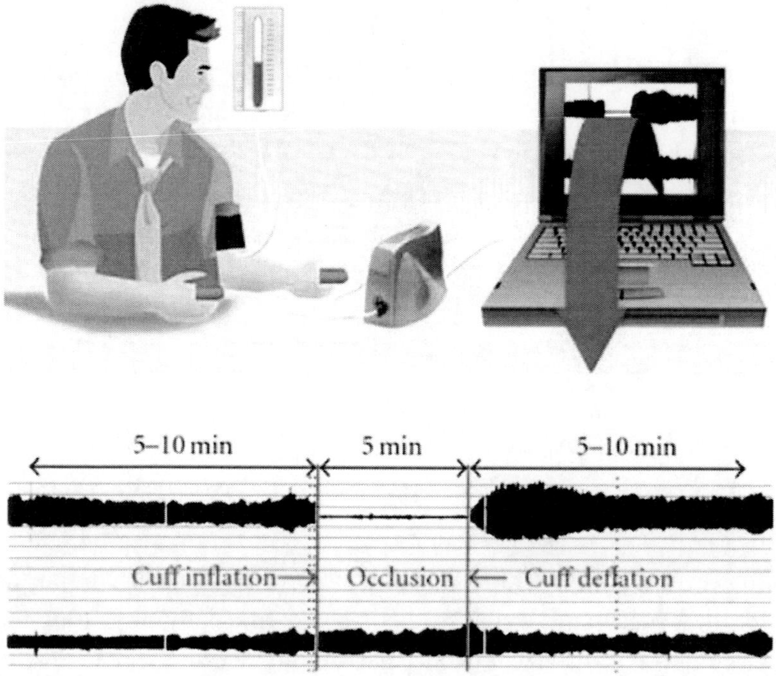

Figure 4. Representation of the modality of execution of an exam with endoPAT. Rev Esp Cardiol. 2012;65:80.

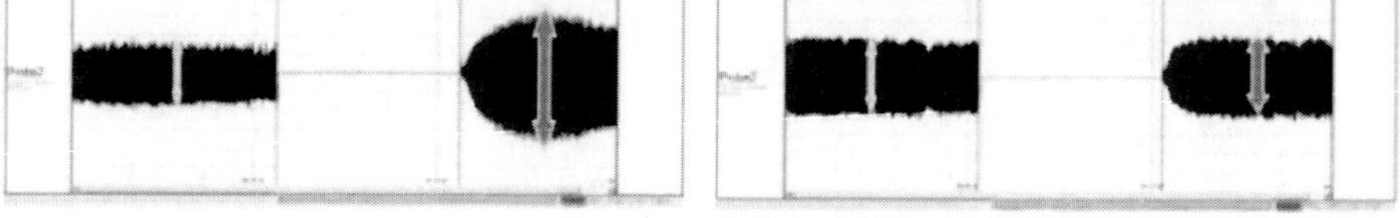

Figure 5. Comparison between a normal (left) and an endothelial dysfunction PAT (right), without signal increase after deflation of the cuff.

An index of 1.67 or below indicates an endothelial dysfunction [54, 56].

According to other authors, also an RHI below 2.0 is considered as dysfunction, whereas an index above this limit is considered to reflect normal endothelial function [55].

It has been demonstrated in several studies that endothelial dysfunction measured with PAT represents a parameter to assess cardiovascular risk in healthy subjects and predicts the risk of further cardiovascular events in patients with CAD [57-64].

4. PAT and FMD, Two Methods Two Disease (Macro and Microvascular Dysfunction)

In the evaluation of endothelial function, it is of primary importance to consider the vascular district studied, since the pathophysiology of the microcirculation is different from that of the resistance vessels (macro-circulation).

These differences could be explained by the different role of NO in the two vascular districts; in microcirculation NO primarily modulates tissue metabolism, while in macro-circulation it is secreted in response to various stimuli [65].

Meta-analysis have compared PAT and FMD showing them having discordant results but similar correlation with cardiovascular outcomes [60, 66].

Indeed, the studies that have used these techniques have shown that they actually investigate the two different vascular districts described above: FMD reflects macrovascular function, while PAT microvascular function. [57, 67-70]

As proof of this, FMD seems to be particularly impaired by traditional risk factors (e.g., age, hypertension), while the peripheral arterial tonometry reactive hyperemia index is more sensitive to metabolic risk factors, especially body mass index and diabetes [59, 60].

In particular, evidence showed that macrovascular endothelial function might be more important in patients with existing atherosclerosis (and so in secondary prevention) and microvascular function might be more important in subclinical dysfunction (like in the younger or adult subjects apparently healthy); in other words, microvascular function may be an earlier indicator of risk.

Thus microvascular and macrovascular function may give important extra information, above and beyond traditional risk factors, in certain situations.

Given that macrovascular and microvascular endothelium are susceptible to different risk factors, whenever possible should be both evaluated.

Moreover the fact that micro- and macro-vascular endothelial function only show a weak correlation with each other should caution against the extrapolation of findings in one circulation level to the other [60].

5. Clinical Relevance of Endotelial Function Assessment

5.1. Endothelial Function as a Marker for Cardiovascular Risk in Primary Prevention

Endothelial dysfunction is not only associated with blown atherosclerosis and cardiovascular disease, but also with every condition predisposing to them (a sort of "risk of developing risk factors") [71]. For example, endothelial dysfunction has been observed in patients with arterial hypertension [72–74], in normotensive subjects with a family history of hypertension, [75] in smokers [76-77], in dyslipidemia [78-79], in ageing [73], diabetes mellitus [80-83], in obesity [83], in hyperhomocysteinemia [84-85], and in patients with inflammatory or infectious diseases [86–88]. Thus, endothelial dysfunction may represent the effect of these risk factors on vascular health, both in peripheral (microvascular and macrovascular) and coronary district [58, 89-90].

So, being endothelial dysfunction an important mechanism for cardiovascular risk, its prognostic value is a logic consequence. The real issue is to understand if measurements of endothelial function could provide more information beyond traditional risk factors and score algorithms to predict CV events in subjects free of cardiovascular or atherosclerotic diseases.

Obviously, in the field of primary prevention it is not possible to consider the use of invasive methods to assess endothelial function, though they have already demonstrated their validity [27, 91].

Several studies have been conducted using noninvasive techniques, in particular FMD and PAT. They demonstrated the value of endothelial function in predicting cardiovascular events, in addition to traditional risk factors, in healthy subjects without heart disease and low clinical risk [57, 92-94].

Some of these studies enrolled a great number of patients [95-96]; for example the Cardiovascular Health Study, in which endothelial dysfunction was evaluated by FMD in healthy subjects aged 72 or more: cardiovascular events were more frequent (in a 5 years follow up) in those with documented endothelial dysfunction, and this correlation was maintained also after adjusting for other risk factors [95].

In this sense, endothelial function was able to add additional information in primary cardiovascular prevention, potentially suggesting that not all individual risk factors have been found yet.

5.2. Endothelial Dysfunction as Prognostic Factor in Patient with Already Established Atherosclerotic Disease

Classically, endothelial function has demonstrated a prognostic value in the field of cardiovascular secondary prevention, namely in those patients with already established coronary artery disease.

Indeed, reduced peripheral endothelial function was demonstrated to be an independent predictor of cardiovascular events in patients with coronary artery disease and acute coronary syndrome [97-98].

Using invasive methods, higher incidences in cardiovascular events was highlighted in patients with non-obstructive coronary artery disease and impaired coronary vascular function [26, 97-100]. In particular, in acute myocardial infarction endothelial dysfunction has been documented to be indicative of a poorer prognosis, especially evaluating microvascular circulation [101-106].

In fact, microvascular dysfunction may contribute to the impaired regulation of myocardial perfusion, leading to myocardial ischemia [107-109]. This acquires particular relevance in presence of mellitus diabetes and others risk factors in the metabolic syndrome [110-113].

Similar results were obtained using noninvasive methods, such as FMD and PAT [97, 98, 100, 114].

Interestingly, it was reported that impaired peripheral endothelial function, measured using RHI, significantly predicts further cardiovascular events independently from coronary plaque complexity assessed by the SYNTAX Score [64].

Moreover, an endothelial dysfunction assessed with FMD has been shown to be an independent predictor of restenosis after single-vessel coronary intervention [115].

It was also demonstrated that endothelial function is an independent predicting factor of 1-year mortality in patients with ischemic advanced heart failure [116].

Interestingly, in heart transplanted patients with graft vasculopathy, endothelial dysfunction is associated with higher progression of coronary intimal thickening and poorer prognosis [117-119].

Therefore, on the basis of the various studies carried out up to now, the prognostic importance of the evaluation of endothelial dysfunction in coronary disease is clear. This, as it will be discussed later, could have important implications from the therapeutic point of view. Indeed, the improvement of peripheral endothelial function seems to be associated with reduction in cardiovascular events [57, 92, 93, 95, 96, 98, 120, 121].

From a pathophysiological point of view, endothelial dysfunction (both in peripheral and coronary arteries) is one of the factors that contributes to the progression of atherosclerosis [49]. Indeed, it has been shown that a greater endothelial dysfunction correlates with the presence of vulnerable atherosclerotic plaques [122]. In particular, it has been evidenced that in these segments there is an imbalance between vasodilator and vasoconstrictor agents, with a reduction of NO activity and an increase in the production of endothelin-1, and that the progression of atherosclerotic process gets more frequently to obstructive artery disease [123, 124].

So measurement of endothelial dysfunction in the setting of secondary prevention may give some important information both in the risk stratification of patients and from a therapeutic point of view.

5.3. Therapeutic Implications

Having widely illustrated the importance of endothelial dysfunction as cardiovascular risk factor and its prognostic value in already established cardiovascular disease, we need to know if there are therapies or other interventions that could improve endothelial function.

Indeed, finding new risk predictor beyond traditional CV risk factors would be useless without the possibility of modifying them directly or indirectly. Moreover, endothelial function could represents a marker to identify responders to therapy and its improvement could be exploited as a therapy target, i.e., an indicator of successful treatment.

Thus the principal questions to answer are:

- What kind of intervention can improve endothelial function?
- Does this improvement of endothelial function always predict a better prognosis for the patient?
- Could endothelial function represent an individual therapeutic target?

Concerning the first question, the possible approaches to act on endothelial dysfunction are both medical/pharmacological and obtained with lifestyle interventions.

Regarding lifestyle approach, many actions demonstrated their benefits on endothelial function: physical exercise [125, 126, 127], weight loss [128–132], dietary modification with a low calories and low fat diet and an increase in foods rich in polyphenols [133–135].

One of the most important intervention is represented by smoking cessation, which determinates great improvement of epicardial coronary endothelial function [76].

The effects of these interventions depend especially on the increase in NO bioavailability, but also on the decrease in the production of endothelium-derived constricting factors, i.e., endothelin-1.

It was demonstrated that cholesterol lowering therapy (statins) improves endothelial function, both in coronary and in peripheral arteries, mostly thanks to their anti-inflammatory and antioxidant properties [136, 137, 138, 139].

Also antihypertensive therapy in general seems to have reversing effects on endothelial dysfunction [140, 141], in particular angiotensin-converting enzyme (ACE)-inhibitors [141, 142, 143, 144, 145], but also others drugs such as angiotensin-receptor blocker (ARBs) [146], calcium channel blockers (CCB) [147-150] and certain β-blockers, in particular the NO-group containing molecule nebivolol [151].

However, there are substances with demonstrated capacity to improve acutely endothelial function that has not proven benefits on morbidity and mortality in patients with cardiovascular disease, for example vitamin C or E as well as folic acid supplementation [152, 153]. This could depend on the dose administrated in the trials conducted or on the presence of other elements of endogenous oxidative stress [154, 155].

Regarding the second question, important studies that have been performed recently [62, 120] have demonstrated that a lack of improvement of endothelial function reflects an increased risk of further cardiovascular events. However, more studies in this respect need to be carried out [156].

The third question reflects a problem still unsolved in the field of cardiovascular therapy. In fact, some patients develop CV events despite an optimized medical therapy (both regarding secondary or primary prevention). Identifying these patients could represent an important challenge in order to implement a therapy that should be as personalized as possible. In this sense, it could be useful to measure the individual impact of therapy on endothelial function, addressing more aggressive therapy in those patients with reduced response.

5.4. Future Perspectives

In the past decade, many studies have suggested that the assessment of endothelial function may provide important information for individual patient risk, progress and guidance of therapy.

Indeed, in addition to being a prognostic factor, the evaluation of endothelial function predicts a better cardiovascular outcome with its own improvement in response to cardio-active therapy [156, 157]. As a consequence, individual endothelial function could be investigated as a therapeutic target. Larger studies in this respect are needed to answer the question whether endothelial function guided therapy helps to improve outcomes.

Regarding primary prevention, the issue is more complex because, as previously discussed, it would be desirable to evaluate endothelial function in patients with a low cardiovascular risk profile in which the traditional elements for the assessment of this CV risk are insufficient [158, 159].

Therefore the role of endothelial function as a predictor of cardiovascular mortality and morbidity should be investigated with targeted and large-scale studies especially in patients who are in the "grey area" of intermediate cardiovascular risk using traditional scores.

Moreover, until now, the studies that used peripheral endothelial function tests showed some limitation: for example most of them enrolled a small number and very selected subgroups of patients; they also required a very long follow up period due to the slow variation in time of the parameters considered by the two techniques.

Further research to evaluate the prognostic utility of both these methods (especially for the more recent PAT) is necessary to compare them with invasive endothelial function test in clinical practice. To now, no evidence support the routine evaluation of endothelial function in patients with or without coronary artery disease. Despite this fact, considering endothelial function both “primum movens” and final target of cardiovascular pathology, we could affirm the role of its functional evaluation to explore “cardiovascular homeostasis” of individual patients. In other terms: the same cardiovascular risk could have different impact in different patients (genetic predisposition? Other unknown risk factors?). Evaluating serially the same parameters in the same patients could allow to recognize the real CV risk profile to optimize and individualize the better therapeutic interventions.

REFERENCES

[1] Noninvasive assessment of endothelial function: the classic methods and the new peripheral arterial tonometry. Vizzardi E1, Gavazzoni M, Della Pina P, Bonadei I, Regazzoni V, Sciatti E, Trichaki E, Raddino R, Metra M. *J Investig Med.* 2014 Aug;62(6):856-64.

[2] Naghavi M, Libby P, Falk E, Casscells SW, Litovsky S, Rumberger J, Badimon JJ, Stefanadis C, Moreno P, Pasterkamp G, Fayad Z, Stone PH, Waxman S, Raggi P, Madjid M, Zarrabi A, Burke A, Yuan C, Fitzgerald PJ, Siscovick DS, de Korte CL, Aikawa M, Juhani Airaksinen KE, Assmann G, Becker CR, Chesebro JH, Farb A, Galis ZS, Jackson C, Jang IK, Koenig W, Lodder RA, March K, Demirovic J, Navab M, Priori SG, Rekhter MD, Bahr R, S. M. G, Mehran R, Colombo A, Boerwinkle E, Ballantyne C, Insull W, Schwartz RS, Vogel R, Serruys PW, Hansson GK, Faxon DP, Kaul S, Drexler H, Greenland P, Muller JE, Virmani R, Ridker PM,

Zipes DP, Shah PK, Willerson JT. From vulnerable plaque to vulnerable patient: a call for new definitions and risk assessment strategies: part II. *Circulation.* 2003;108:1772–1778.

[3] Johnson KM, Dowe DA, Brink JA. Traditional clinical risk assessment tools do not accurately predict coronary atherosclerotic plaque burden: a CT angiography study. *Am J Roentgenol.* 2009;192:235–243.

[4] Naghavi M, Libby P, Falk E, Casscells SW, Litovsky S, Rumberger J, Badimon JJ, Stefanadis C, Moreno P, Pasterkamp G, Fayad Z, Stone PH, Waxman S, Raggi P, Madjid M, Zarrabi A, Burke A, Yuan C, Fitzgerald PJ, Siscovick DS, de Korte CL, Aikawa M, Juhani Airaksinen KE, Assmann G, Becker CR, Chesebro JH, Farb A, Galis ZS, Jackson C, Jang IK, Koenig W, Lodder RA, March K, Demirovic J, Navab M, Priori SG, Rekhter MD, Bahr R, Grundy SM, Mehran R, Colombo A, Boerwinkle E, Ballantyne C, Insull W Jr, Schwartz RS, Vogel R, Serruys PW, Hansson GK, Faxon DP, Kaul S, Drexler H, Greenland P, Muller JE, Virmani R, Ridker PM, Zipes DP, Shah PK, Willerson JT. From vulnerable plaque to vulnerable patient: a call for new definitions and risk assessment strategies: part I. *Circulation.* 2003;108:1664–1672.

[5] Schechter AN, Gladwin MT. Hemoglobin and the paracrine and endocrine functions of nitric oxide. *N Engl J Med.* 2003; 348: 1483–1485.

[6] Furchgott RF, Zawadzki JV. The obligatory role of endothelial cells in the relaxation of arterial smooth muscle by acetylcholine. Nature. 1980; 288: 373–376. *Nature.* 1980 Nov 27;288(5789):373-6.

[7] Endothelium-derived relaxing factor: discovery, early studies, and identification as nitric oxide. Furchgott RF1. *Biosci Rep.* 1999 Aug;19(4):235-51.

[8] Corson MA, James NL, Latta SE, Nerem RM, Berk BC, Harrison DG. Phosphorylation of endothelial nitric oxide synthase in response to fluid shear stress. *Circ Res*. 1996; 79: 984–991.

[9] Saye JA, Singer HA, Peach MJ. Role of endothelium in conversion of angiotensin I to angiotensin II in rabbit aorta. *Hypertension.* 1984; 6: 216–221.

[10] Kinlay S, Behrendt D, Wainstein M, Beltrame J, Fang JC, Creager MA, Selwyn AP, Ganz P. Role of endothelin-1 in the active constriction of human atherosclerotic coronary arteries. *Circulation.* 2001; 104: 1114–1118.

[11] Patten RD, Konstam MA. *Ventricular remodeling and the renin angiotensin aldosterone system.*

[12] Walmor C. De Mello, A. H. Jan Danser. *Angiotensin II and the Heart.*

[13] Ghosh S, Karin M. Missing pieces in the NF-κB puzzle. *Cell.* 2002; 109: S81–S96.

[14] Anderson 1999 *Assessment and treatment of endothelial dysfunction in humans.*

[15] Radomski MW, Palmer RM, Moncada S. *The anti-aggregating properties of vascular endothelium: interactions between prostacyclin and nitric oxide.*

[16] Mooren OL, Li J, Nawas J, Cooper JA. *Endothelial cells use dynamic actin to facilitate lymphocyte transendothelial migration and maintain the monolayer barrier.*

[17] Peiró C, Redondo J, Rodríguez-Martínez MA, Angulo J, Marín J, Sánchez-Ferrer CF. *Influence of endothelium on cultured vascular smooth muscle cell proliferation.*

[18] Coronary endothelial function assessment using self-gated cardiac cine MRI and k-t sparse SENSE. Yerly J, Ginami G, Nordio G, Coristine AJ, Coppo S, Monney P, Stuber M. *Magn Reson Med.* 2016 Nov;76(5):1443-1454. doi: 10.1002/mrm.26050. Epub 2015 Nov 24.

[19] Self-gated golden angle spiral cine MRI for coronary endothelial function assessment. Bonanno G, Hays AG, Weiss RG, Schär M. *Magn Reson Med.* 2017 Dec 27. doi: 10.1002/mrm.27060. [Epub ahead of print].

[20] Quantitative CMR markers of impaired vascular reactivity associated with age and peripheral artery disease. Langham MC1, Englund EK, Mohler ER 3rd, Li C, Rodgers ZB, Floyd TF, Wehrli FW. *J Cardiovasc Magn Reson.* 2013 Feb 13;15:17. doi: 10.1186/1532-429X-15-17.

[21] Coronary endothelial function assessment using self-gated cardiac cine MRI and k-t sparse SENSE. Yerly J, Ginami G, Nordio G, Coristine AJ, Coppo S, Monney P, Stuber M. *Magn Reson Med.* 2016 Nov;76(5):1443-1454. doi: 10.1002/mrm.26050. Epub 2015 Nov 24.

[22] Impact of cardiac magnetic resonance on endothelial function in type 2 diabetic patients. Xiang G, Xiang L, He H, Zhang J, Dong J. *Atherosclerosis.* 2015 Mar; 239(1):131-6. doi: 10.1016/ j.atherosclerosis.2014.12.028. Epub 2015 Jan 13.

[23] Effects of age and smoking on endothelial function assessed by quantitative cardiovascular magnetic resonance in the peripheral and central vasculature. Langham MC, Zhou Y, Chirico EN, Magland JF, Sehgal CM, Englund EK, Mohler ER 3rd, Guo W8, Barhoum S9, Wehrli FW10. *J Cardiovasc Magn Reson.* 2015 Feb 19;17:19. doi: 10.1186/s12968-015-0110-8.

[24] Flammer AJ, Anderson T, Celermajer DS, et al. The assessment of endothelial function: from research into clinical practice. *Circulation.* 2012; 126:753–767. [PubMed: 22869857].

[25] Ludmer PL, Selwyn AP, Shook TL, et al. Paradoxical vasoconstriction induced by acetylcholine in atherosclerotic coronary arteries. *The New England journal of medicine.* 1986; 315:1046–1051. [PubMed: 3093861]

[26] Schachinger V, Britten MB, Zeiher AM. Prognostic impact of coronary vasodilator dysfunction on adverse long-term outcome of coronary heart disease. *Circulation.* 2000; 101:1899–1906. [PubMed: 10779454].

[27] Halcox JP, Schenke WH, Zalos G, et al. Prognostic value of coronary vascular endothelial dysfunction. *Circulation.* 2002; 106:653–658. [PubMed: 12163423]

[28] Targonski PV, Bonetti PO, Pumper GM, Higano ST, Holmes DR Jr, Lerman A. Coronary endothelial dysfunction is associated with an increased risk of cerebrovascular events. *Circulation.* 2003; 107:2805–2809. [PubMed: 12771004].

[29] Yoon MH, Reriani M, Mario G, et al. Long-term endothelin receptor antagonism attenuates coronary plaque progression in patients with early atherosclerosis. *International journal of cardiology.* 2013; 168:1316–1321. [PubMed: 23290081].

[30] Joannides R, Haefeli WE, Linder L, Richard V, Bakkali EH, Thuillez C, Lüscher TF. Nitric oxide is responsible for flow-dependent dilatation of human peripheral conduit arteries *in vivo. Circulation.* 1995; 91:1314–1319. [PubMed: 7867167].

[31] Lieberman EH, Gerhard MD, Uehata A, Selwyn AP, Ganz P, Yeung AC, Creager MA. Flowinduced vasodilation of the human brachial artery is impaired in patients <40 years of age with coronary artery disease. *The American journal of cardiology.* 1996; 78:1210–1214. [PubMed: 8960576].

[32] Joannides R, Richard V, Haefeli WE, Linder L, Lüscher TF, Thuillez C. Role of basal and stimulated release of nitric oxide in the regulation of radial artery caliber in humans. *Hypertension.* 1995; 26:327–331. [PubMed: 7635543].

[33] Parker BA, Tschakovsky ME, Augeri AL, Polk DM, Thompson PD, Kiernan FJ. Heterogenous vasodilator pathways underlie flow-mediated dilation in men and women. *American journal of physiology.* 2011; 301:H1118–1126. [PubMed: 21642502].

[34] Charakida M, Masi S, Luscher TF, Kastelein JJ, Deanfield JE. Assessment of atherosclerosis: the role of flow-mediated dilatation. *European heart journal.* 2010; 31:2854–2861. [PubMed: 20864485].

[35] Harris RA, Nishiyama SK, Wray DW, Richardson RS. Ultrasound assessment of flow-mediated dilation. *Hypertension.* 2010; 55:1075–1085. [PubMed: 20351340]

[36] Thijssen DH, Black MA, Pyke KE, Padilla J, Atkinson G, Harris RA, Parker B, Widlansky ME, Tschakovsky ME, Green DJ.

Assessment of flow-mediated dilation in humans: a methodological and physiological guideline. *American journal of physiology*. 2011; 300:H2–12. [PubMed: 20952670].

[37] Corretti MC, Anderson TJ, Benjamin EJ, Celermajer D, Charbonneau F, Creager MA, Deanfield J, Drexler H, Gerhard-Herman M, Herrington D, Vallance P, Vita J, Vogel R. Guidelines for the ultrasound assessment of endothelial-dependent flow-mediated vasodilation of the brachial artery: a report of the International Brachial Artery Reactivity Task Force. *Journal of the American College of Cardiology*. 2002; 39:257–265. [PubMed: 11788217].

[38] Deanfield J, Donald A, Ferri C, Giannattasio C, Halcox J, Halligan S, Lerman A, Mancia G, Oliver JJ, Pessina AC, Rizzoni D, Rossi GP, Salvetti A, Schiffrin EL, Taddei S, Webb DJ. 8. Part I: Methodological issues for assessment in the different vascular beds: a statement by the Working Group on Endothelin and Endothelial Factors of the European Society of Hypertension. *J Hypertens*. 2005; 23:7–17. [PubMed: 15643116].

[39] Donald AE, Halcox JP, Charakida M, Storry C, Wallace SM, Cole TJ, Friberg P, Deanfield JE. Methodological approaches to optimize reproducibility and power in clinical studies of flowmediated dilation. *Journal of the American College of Cardiology*. 2008; 51:1959–1964. [PubMed: 18482664].

[40] Celermajer DS, Sorensen KE, Bull C, Robinson J, Deanfield JE. Endothelium-dependent dilation in the systemic arteries of asymptomatic subjects relates to coronary risk factors and their interaction. *J Am Coll Cardiol*. 1994; 24:1468-1474.

[41] Black MA, Cable NT, Thijssen DH, Green DJ. Importance of measuring the time course of flow-mediated dilation in humans. *Hypertension*. 2008; 51: 203-210.

[42] Dyson KS, Argarwal N, Williams-Bell M, Bhatti A, Denniss SG, Hughson RL. Sustained hyperaemia stimulus is necessary to induce flow-mediated dilation of the human brachial artery. *Clin Physiol Funct Imaging*. 2011; 31: 415-421.

[43] Liuni A, Luca MC, Lisi M, Dragoni S, Di Stolfo G, Mariani JA, Uxa A, Gori T, Parker JD. Observations of time-based measures of flow-mediated dilation of forearm conduit arteries: implications for the accurate assessment of endothelial function. *Am J Physiol Heart Circ Physiol*. 2010; 299: H939-945.

[44] Betik AC, Luckham VB, Hughson RL. Flow-mediated dilation in human brachial artery after different circulatory occlusion conditions. *Am J Physiol Heart Circ Physiol.* 2004; 286: H442-448.

[45] Strisciuglio, Teresa; Luca, Stefania De; Capuano, Ernesto; Luciano, Rossella; Niglio, Tullio; Trimarco, Bruno; Galasso, Gennaro (2014-06-01). "Endothelial Dysfunction: Its Clinical Value and Methods of Assessment." *Current Atherosclerosis Reports*. 16 (6): 417. doi:10.1007/s11883-014-0417-1. ISSN 1523-3804).

[46] Inaba Y, Chen JA, Bergmann SR. Prediction of future cardiovascular outcomes by flow-mediated vasodilatation of brachial artery: a meta-analysis. *The international journal of cardiovascular imaging.* 2010; 26:631–640. [PubMed: 20339920].

[47] Lekakis J, Abraham P, Balbarini A, Blann A, Boulanger CM, Cockcroft J, Cosentino F, Deanfield J, Gallino A, Ikonomidis I, Kremastinos D, Landmesser U, Protogerou A, Stefanadis C, Tousoulis D, Vassalli G, Vink H, Werner N, Wilkinson I, Vlachopoulos C. Methods for evaluating endothelial function: a position statement from the European Society of Cardiology Working Group on Peripheral Circulation. *Eur J Cardiovasc Prev Rehabil.* 2011;18(6):775-89.

[48] Yan RT, Anderson TJ, Charbonneau F, Title L, Verma S, Lonn E. Relationship between carotid artery intima-media thickness and brachial artery flow-mediated dilation in middle-aged healthy men. *Journal of the American College of Cardiology*. 2005; 45:1980–1986. [PubMed: 15963396].

[49] Halcox JP, Donald AE, Ellins E, Witte DR, Shipley MJ, Brunner EJ, Marmot MG, Deanfield JE. Endothelial function predicts progression of carotid intima-media thickness. *Circulation*. 2009; 119:1005–1012. [PubMed: 19204308].

[50] Gori T, Grotti S, Dragoni S, Lisi M, Di Stolfo G, Sonnati S, Fineschi M, Parker JD. Assessment of vascular function: flow-mediated constriction complements the information of flow-mediated dilatation. *Heart* (British Cardiac Society). 2010; 96:141–147. [PubMed: 19858140].

[51] Gori T, Dragoni S, Lisi M, Di Stolfo G, Sonnati S, Fineschi M, Parker JD. Conduit artery constriction mediated by low flow a novel noninvasive method for the assessment of vascular function. *Journal of the American College of Cardiology*. 2008; 51:1953–1958. [PubMed: 18482663].

[52] Bellien J, Joannides R, Iacob M, Arnaud P, Thuillez C. Evidence for a basal release of a cytochrome-related endothelium-derived hyperpolarizing factor in the radial artery in humans. *Am J Physiol Heart Circ Physiol*. 2006; 290: H1347-1352.

[53] Evaluation of endothelial function by peripheral arterial tonometry and relation with the nitric oxide pathway. Hedetoft M, Olsen NV. *Nitric Oxide*. 2014 Nov 15;42:1-8. doi: 10.1016/j.niox.2014.07.003. Epub 2014 Jul 23.

[54] Noninvasive identification of patients with early coronary atherosclerosis by assessment of digital reactive hyperemia. Bonetti PO, Pumper GM, Higano ST, Holmes DR, Jr, Kuvin JT, Lerman A. *J Am Coll Cardiol.* 2004;44:2137–2141.

[55] Endothelial function in a cardiovascular risk population with borderline ankle–brachial index. Kari Syvänen, Päivi Korhonen, Auli Partanen, and Pertti Aarnio. *Vasc Health Risk Manag*. 2011;7: 97–101.

[56] Reproducibility of peripheral arterial tonometry measurements in male cardiovascular patients. Nil M1, Schäfer D, Radtke T, Saner H, Wilhelm M, Eser P. *Eur J Clin Invest*. 2014 Nov;44(11):1065-71. doi: 10.1111/eci.12341.

[57] Rubinshtein R, Kuvin JT, Soffler M, et al. Assessment of endothelial function by non-invasive peripheral arterial tonometry predicts late cardiovascular adverse events. *European heart journal*. 2010; 31:1142–1148. [PubMed: 20181680].

[58] Bonetti PO, Pumper GM, Higano ST, Holmes DR Jr, Kuvin JT, Lerman A. Noninvasive identification of patients with early coronary atherosclerosis by assessment of digital reactive hyperemia. *Journal of the American College of Cardiology*. 2004; 44:2137–2141. [PubMed: 15582310].

[59] Hamburg NM, Keyes MJ, Larson MG, Vasan RS, Schnabel R, Pryde MM, Mitchell GF, Sheffy J, Vita JA, Benjamin EJ. Cross-sectional relations of digital vascular function to cardiovascular risk factors in the Framingham Heart Study. *Circulation*. 2008; 117:2467–2474. [PubMed: 18458169].

[60] Hamburg NM, Palmisano J, Larson MG, Sullivan LM, Lehman BT, Vasan RS, Levy D, Mitchell GF, Vita JA, Benjamin EJ. Relation of brachial and digital measures of vascular function in the community: the Framingham heart study. *Hypertension*. 2011; 57:390–396. [PubMed: 21263120].

[61] Schnabel RB, Schulz A, Wild PS, Sinning CR, Wilde S, Eleftheriadis M, Herkenhoff S, Zeller T, Lubos E, Lackner KJ, Warnholtz A, Gori T, Blankenberg S, Munzel T. Noninvasive vascular function measurement in the community: cross-sectional relations and comparison of methods. *Circ Cardiovasc Imaging*. 2011; 4:371–380. [PubMed: 21551420].

[62] Modena MG, Bonetti L, Coppi F, Bursi F, Rossi R. Prognostic role of reversible endothelial dysfunction in hypertensive postmenopausal women. *Journal of the American College of Cardiology*. 2002; 40:505–510. [PubMed: 12142118].

[63] Xu Y, Arora RC, Hiebert BM, et al. Non-invasive endothelial function testing and the risk of adverse outcomes: a *systematic review and meta-analysis. European* heart journal cardiovascular *Imaging*. 2014; 15:736–746. [PubMed: 24399339].

[64] Matsuzawa Y, Sugiyama S, Sumida H, et al. Peripheral endothelial function and cardiovascular events in high-risk patients. *Journal of the American Heart Association*. 2013; 2:e000426. [PubMed: 24275629].

[65] Trochu JN, Bouhour JB, Kaley G, Hintze TH. Role of endothelium-derived nitric oxide in the regulation of cardiac oxygen metabolism: implications in health and disease. *Circulation research.* 2000; 87:1108–1117. [PubMed: 11110767].

[66] Prognostic Value of Flow-Mediated Vasodilation in Brachial Artery and Fingertip Artery for Cardiovascular Events: A Systematic Review and Meta-Analysis. Matsuzawa Y, Kwon TG, Lennon RJ, Lerman LO, Lerman A. *J Am Heart Assoc*. 2015 Nov 13;4(11). pii: e002270. doi: 10.1161/JAHA.115.002270.

[67] Anderson TJ, Charbonneau F, Title LM, Buithieu J, Rose MS, Conradson H, Hildebrand K, Fung M, Verma S, Lonn EM. Microvascular function predicts cardiovascular events in primary prevention: long-term results from the Firefighters and Their Endothelium (FATE) study. *Circulation.* 2011; 123:163–169. [PubMed: 21200002].

[68] Lind L, Berglund L, Larsson A, Sundstrom J. Endothelial function in resistance and conduit arteries and 5-year risk of cardiovascular disease. *Circulation*. 2011; 123:1545–1551. [PubMed: 21444885].

[69] Matsuzawa Y, Sugiyama S, Sugamura K, Nozaki T, Ohba K, Konishi M, Matsubara J, Sumida H, Kaikita K, Kojima S, Nagayoshi Y, Yamamuro M, Izumiya Y, Iwashita S, Matsui K, Jinnouchi H, Kimura K, Umemura S, Ogawa H. Digital assessment of endothelial function and ischemic heart disease in women. *Journal of the American College of Cardiology.* 2010; 55:1688–1696. [PubMed: 20394872].

[70] [*Assessment of endothelial dysfunction for prevention of complications in patients with lesions of peripheral arteries*]. [Article in Russian; Abstract available in Russian from the publisher]. Pokrovskiĭ AV, Kul'bak VA, Kremenchugskaia TA, Fedorov EE. Angiol Sosud Khir. 2017;23(4):29-34.

[71] Brunner H, Cockcroft JR, Deanfield J, Donald A, Ferrannini E, Halcox J, Kiowski W, Luscher TF, Mancia G, Natali A, Oliver JJ, Pessina AC, Rizzoni D, Rossi GP, Salvetti A, Spieker LE, Taddei S, Webb DJ. Endothelial function and dysfunction. Part II:

Association with cardiovascular risk factors and diseases. A statement by the Working Group on Endothelins and Endothelial Factors of the European Society of Hypertension. *J Hypertens*. 2005; 23:233–246. [PubMed: 15662207].

[72] Panza JA, Quyyumi AA, Brush JJ, Epstein SE. Abnormal endothelium-dependent vascular relaxation in patients with essential hypertension. *The New England journal of medicine*. 1990; 323:22–27. [PubMed: 2355955].

[73] Linder L, Kiowski W, Buhler FR, Luscher TF. Indirect evidence for release of endotheliumderived relaxing factor in human forearm circulation *in vivo*. Blunted response in essential hypertension. *Circulation*. 1990; 81:1762–1767. [PubMed: 2344673].

[74] Treasure CB, Manoukian SV, Klein JL, Vita JA, Nabel EG, Renwick GH, Selwyn AP, Alexander RW, Ganz P. Epicardial coronary artery responses to acetylcholine are impaired in hypertensive patients. *Circulation research*. 1992; 71:776–781. [PubMed: 1516154].

[75] Taddei S, Virdis A, Mattei P, Ghiadoni L, Sudano I, Salvetti A. Defective L-arginine-nitric oxide pathway in offspring of essential hypertensive patients. *Circulation*. 1996; 94:1298–1303. [PubMed: 8822983].

[76] Celermajer DS, Sorensen KE, Georgakopoulos D, Bull C, Thomas O, Robinson J, Deanfield JE. Cigarette smoking is associated with dose-related and potentially reversible impairment of endothelium-dependent dilation in healthy young adults. *Circulation*. 1993; 88:2149–2155. [PubMed: 8222109].

[77] Zeiher AM, Schachinger V, Minners J. Long-term cigarette smoking impairs endotheliumdependent coronary arterial vasodilator function. *Circulation*. 1995; 92:1094–1100. [PubMed: 7648652].

[78] a. Casino PR, Kilcoyne CM, Quyyumi AA, Hoeg JM, Panza JA. The role of nitric oxide in endothelium-dependent vasodilation of hypercholesterolemic patients. *Circulation*. 1993; 88:2541–2547. [PubMed: 8252665] Makimattila S, Virkamaki A, Groop PH,

Cockcroft J, Utriainen T, Fagerudd J, Yki-Jarvinen H. Chronic hyperglycemia impairs endothelial function and insulin sensitivity via different mechanisms in insulin-dependent diabetes mellitus. *Circulation*. 1996; 94:1276–1282. [PubMed: 8822980]. b. Spieker LE, Sudano I, Hurlimann D, Lerch PG, Lang MG, Binggeli C, Corti R, Ruschitzka F, Luscher TF, Noll G. High-density lipoprotein restores endothelial function in hypercholesterolemic men. *Circulation*. 2002; 105:1399–1402. [PubMed: 11914243].

[79] Calver A, Collier J, Vallance P. Inhibition and stimulation of nitric oxide synthesis in the human forearm arterial bed of patients with insulin-dependent diabetes. *J Clin Invest*. 1992; 90:2548– 2554. [PubMed: 1469103].

[80] Cosentino F, Eto M, De Paolis P, van der Loo B, Bachschmid M, Ullrich V, Kouroedov A, Delli Gatti C, Joch H, Volpe M, Luscher TF. High glucose causes upregulation of cyclooxygenase-2 and alters prostanoid profile in human endothelial cells: role of protein kinase C and reactive oxygen species. *Circulation*. 2003; 107:1017–1023. [PubMed: 12600916].

[81] Smits P, Kapma JA, Jacobs MC, Lutterman J, Thien T. Endothelium-dependent vascular relaxation in patients with type I diabetes. *Diabetes*. 1993; 42:148–153. [PubMed: 8420811].

[82] Steinberg HO, Chaker H, Leaming R, Johnson A, Brechtel G, Baron AD. Obesity/insulin resistance is associated with endothelial dysfunction. Implications for the syndrome of insulin resistance. *J Clin Invest*. 1996; 97:2601–2610. [PubMed: 8647954].

[83] Virdis A, Ghiadoni L, Cardinal H, Favilla S, Duranti P, Birindelli R, Magagna A, Bernini G, Salvetti G, Taddei S, Salvetti A. Mechanisms responsible for endothelial dysfunction induced by fasting hyperhomocystinemia in normotensive subjects and patients with essential hypertension. *Journal of the American College of Cardiology*. 2001; 38:1106–1115. [PubMed: 11583890].

[84] Tawakol A, Forgione MA, Stuehlinger M, Alpert NM, Cooke JP, Loscalzo J, Fischman AJ, Creager MA, Gewirtz H. Homocysteine impairs coronary microvascular dilator function in humans. *Journal*

of the American College of Cardiology. 2002; 40:1051–1058. [PubMed: 12354427].

[85] Hurlimann D, Forster A, Noll G, Enseleit F, Chenevard R, Distler O, Bechir M, Spieker LE, Neidhart M, Michel BA, Gay RE, Luscher TF, Gay S, Ruschitzka F. Anti-tumor necrosis factoralpha treatment improves endothelial function in patients with rheumatoid arthritis. *Circulation*. 2002; 106:2184–2187. [PubMed: 12390945].

[86] Flammer AJ, Vo NT, Ledergerber B, Hermann F, Gamperli A, Huttner A, Evison J, Baumgartner I, Cavassini M, Hayoz D, Quitzau K, Hersberger M, Sudano I, Ruschitzka F, Luscher TF, Noll G, Weber R. Effect of atazanavir versus other protease inhibitor-containing antiretroviral therapy on endothelial function in HIV-infected persons: randomised controlled trial. *Heart* (British Cardiac Society). 2009; 95:385–390. [PubMed: 18653575].

[87] Flammer AJ, Sudano I, Hermann F, Gay S, Forster A, Neidhart M, Kunzler P, Enseleit F, Periat D, Hermann M, Nussberger J, Luscher TF, Corti R, Noll G, Ruschitzka F. Angiotensin-converting enzyme inhibition improves vascular function in rheumatoid arthritis. *Circulation*. 2008; 117:2262–2269. [PubMed: 18427133].

[88] Anderson TJ, Uehata A, Gerhard MD, Meredith IT, Knab S, Delagrage D, Lieberman EH, Ganz P, Creager MA, Yeung AC, Selwyn AP. Close relation of endothelial function in the human coronary and peripheral circulation. *Journal of the American College of Cardiology*. 1995; 26:1235–1241. [PubMed: 7594037].

[89] Takase B, Uehata A, Akima T, Nagai T, Nishioka T, Hamabe A, Satomura K, Ohsuzu F, Kurita A. Endothelium-dependent flow-mediated vasodilation in coronary and brachial arteries in suspected coronary artery disease. *The American journal of cardiology*. 1998; 82:1535–1539. A1537–1538. [PubMed: 9874063].

[90] Schindler TH, Hornig B, Buser PT, Olschewski M, Magosaki N, Pfisterer M, Nitzsche EU, Solzbach U, Just H. Prognostic value of abnormal vasoreactivity of epicardial coronary arteries to sympathetic stimulation in patients with normal coronary

angiograms. *Arteriosclerosis, thrombosis, and vascular biology.* 2003; 23:495–501.

[91] Shechter M, Issachar A, Marai I, Koren-Morag N, Freinark D, Shahar Y, Shechter A, Feinberg MS. Long-term association of brachial artery flow-mediated vasodilation and cardiovascular events in middle-aged subjects with no apparent heart disease. *Int J Cardiol.* 2009; 134:52–58. [PubMed: 18479768].

[92] Hirsch L, Shechter A, Feinberg MS, Koren-Morag N, Shechter M. The impact of early compared to late morning hours on brachial endothelial function and long-term cardiovascular events in healthy subjects with no apparent coronary heart disease. *Int J Cardiol.* 2011; 151:342–347. [PubMed: 20832878].

[93] Rossi R, Nuzzo A, Origliani G, Modena MG. Prognostic role of flow-mediated dilation and cardiac risk factors in post-menopausal women. *Journal of the American College of Cardiology.* 2008; 51:997–1002. [PubMed: 18325438].

[94] Yeboah J, Crouse JR, Hsu FC, Burke GL, Herrington DM. Brachial flow-mediated dilation predicts incident cardiovascular events in older adults: the Cardiovascular Health Study. *Circulation.* 2007; 115:2390–2397. [PubMed: 17452608].

[95] Yeboah J, Folsom AR, Burke GL, Johnson C, Polak JF, Post W, Lima JA, Crouse JR, Herrington DM. Predictive value of brachial flow-mediated dilation for incident cardiovascular events in a population-based study: the multi-ethnic study of atherosclerosis. *Circulation.* 2009; 120:502–509. [PubMed: 19635967].

[96] Heitzer T, Schlinzig T, Krohn K, Meinertz T, Munzel T. Endothelial dysfunction, oxidative stress, and risk of cardiovascular events in patients with coronary artery disease. *Circulation.* 2001; 104:2673–2678. [PubMed: 11723017].

[97] Fichtlscherer S, Breuer S, Zeiher AM. Prognostic value of systemic endothelial dysfunction in patients with acute coronary syndromes: further evidence for the existence of the “vulnerable” patient. *Circulation.* 2004; 110:1926–1932. [PubMed: 15451794].

[98] Suwaidi JA, Hamasaki S, Higano ST, Nishimura RA, Holmes DR Jr, Lerman A. Long-term follow-up of patients with mild coronary artery disease and endothelial dysfunction. *Circulation.* 2000; 101:948–954. [PubMed: 10704159].

[99] Lerman A, Zeiher AM. Endothelial function: cardiac events. *Circulation.* 2005; 111:363–368. [PubMed: 15668353].

[100] Morishima I, Sone T, Okumura K, Tsuboi H, Kondo J, Mukawa H, Matsui H, Toki Y, Ito T, Hayakawa T. Angiographic no-reflow phenomenon as a predictor of adverse long-term outcome in patients treated with percutaneous transluminal coronary angioplasty for first acute myocardial infarction. *Journal of the American College of Cardiology.* 2000; 36:1202–1209. [PubMed: 11028471].

[101] Sorajja P, Gersh BJ, Costantini C, McLaughlin MG, Zimetbaum P, Cox DA, Garcia E, Tcheng JE, Mehran R, Lansky AJ, Kandzari DE, Grines CL, Stone GW. Combined prognostic utility of ST-segment recovery and myocardial blush after primary percutaneous coronary intervention in acute myocardial infarction. *European heart journal.* 2005; 26:667–674. [PubMed: 15734768].

[102] Wu KC, Zerhouni EA, Judd RM, Lugo-Olivieri CH, Barouch LA, Schulman SP, Blumenthal RS, Lima JA. Prognostic significance of microvascular obstruction by magnetic resonance imaging in patients with acute myocardial infarction. *Circulation.* 1998; 97:765–772. [PubMed: 9498540].

[103] Prasad A, Stone GW, Aymong E, Zimetbaum PJ, McLaughlin M, Mehran R, Garcia E, Tcheng JE, Cox DA, Grines CL, Gersh BJ. Impact of ST-segment resolution after primary angioplasty on outcomes after myocardial infarction in elderly patients: an analysis from the CADILLAC trial. *American heart journal.* 2004; 147:669–675. [PubMed: 15077083].

[104] Ndrepepa G, Tiroch K, Fusaro M, Keta D, Seyfarth M, Byrne RA, Pache J, Alger P, Mehilli J, Schomig A, Kastrati A. 5-year prognostic value of no-reflow phenomenon after percutaneous coronary intervention in patients with acute myocardial infarction.

Journal of the American College of Cardiology. 2010; 55:2383–2389. [PubMed: 20488311].

[105] Galiuto L, Lombardo A, Maseri A, Santoro L, Porto I, Cianflone D, Rebuzzi AG, Crea F. Temporal evolution and functional outcome of no reflow: sustained and spontaneously reversible patterns following successful coronary recanalisation. *Heart* (British Cardiac Society). 2003; 89:731–737. [PubMed: 12807843].

[106] Hasdai D, Gibbons RJ, Holmes DR Jr, Higano ST, Lerman A. Coronary endothelial dysfunction in humans is associated with myocardial perfusion defects. *Circulation.* 1997; 96:3390–3395. [PubMed: 9396432].

[107] Lerman A, Holmes DR, Herrmann J, Gersh BJ. Microcirculatory dysfunction in ST-elevation myocardial infarction: cause, consequence, or both? *European heart journal*. 2007; 28:788–797. [PubMed: 17347176].

[108] Albertal M, Voskuil M, Piek JJ, de Bruyne B, Van Langenhove G, Kay PI, Costa MA, Boersma E, Beijsterveldt T, Sousa JE, Belardi JA, Serruys PW. Coronary flow velocity reserve after percutaneous interventions is predictive of periprocedural outcome. *Circulation.* 2002; 105:1573– 1578. [PubMed: 11927525].

[109] Angeja BG, de Lemos J, Murphy SA, Marble SJ, Antman EM, Cannon CP, Braunwald E, Gibson CM. Impact of diabetes mellitus on epicardial and microvascular flow after fibrinolytic therapy. *American heart journal*. 2002; 144:649–656. [PubMed: 12360161].

[110] Kurisu S, Inoue I, Kawagoe T, Ishihara M, Shimatani Y, Nishioka K, Umemura T, Nakamura S, Yoshida M. Diabetes mellitus is associated with insufficient microvascular reperfusion following revascularization for anterior acute myocardial infarction. *Intern Med*. 2003; 42:554–559. [PubMed: 12879945].

[111] Celik T, Turhan H, Kursaklioglu H, Iyisoy A, Yuksel UC, Ozmen N, Isik E. Impact of metabolic syndrome on myocardial perfusion grade after primary percutaneous coronary intervention in patients with acute ST elevation myocardial infarction. *Coronary artery disease*. 2006; 17:339– 343. [PubMed: 16707956].

[112] Clavijo LC, Pinto TL, Kuchulakanti PK, Torguson R, Chu WW, Satler LF, Kent KM, Suddath WO, Pichard AD, Waksman R. Metabolic syndrome in patients with acute myocardial infarction is associated with increased infarct size and inhospital complications. *Cardiovasc Revasc Med*. 2006; 7:7–11. [PubMed: 16513517].

[113] Chan SY, Mancini GB, Kuramoto L, Schulzer M, Frohlich J, Ignaszewski A. The prognostic importance of endothelial dysfunction and carotid atheroma burden in patients with coronary artery disease. *Journal of the American College of Cardiology*. 2003; 42:1037–1043. [PubMed: 13678927].

[114] Patti G, Pasceri V, Melfi R, Goffredo C, Chello M, D'Ambrosio A, Montesanti R, Di Sciascio G. Impaired flow-mediated dilation and risk of restenosis in patients undergoing coronary stent implantation. *Circulation*. 2005; 111:70–75. [PubMed: 15630038].

[115] Shechter M, Matetzky S, Arad M, Feinberg MS, Freimark D. Vascular endothelial function predicts mortality risk in patients with advanced ischaemic chronic heart failure. *Eur J Heart Fail*. 2009; 11:588–593. [PubMed: 19406838].

[116] Davis SF, Yeung AC, Meredith IT, Charbonneau F, Ganz P, Selwyn AP, Anderson TJ. Early endothelial dysfunction predicts the development of transplant coronary artery disease at 1 year posttransplant. *Circulation*. 1996; 93:457–462. [PubMed: 8565162].

[117] Kubrich M, Petrakopoulou P, Kofler S, Nickel T, Kaczmarek I, Meiser BM, Reichart B, von Scheidt W, Weis M. Impact of coronary endothelial dysfunction on adverse long-term outcome after heart transplantation. *Transplantatio*n. 2008; 85:1580–1587. [PubMed: 18551063].

[118] Hollenberg SM, Klein LW, Parrillo JE, Scherer M, Burns D, Tamburro P, Oberoi M, Johnson MR, Costanzo MR. Coronary endothelial dysfunction after heart transplantation predicts allograft vasculopathy and cardiac death. *Circulation*. 2001; 104:3091–3096. [PubMed: 11748106].

[119] Kitta Y, Obata JE, Nakamura T, et al. Persistent impairment of endothelial vasomotor function has a negative impact on outcome in

patients with coronary artery disease. *Journal of the American College of Cardiology*. 2009; 53:323–330. [PubMed: 19161880].

[120] Ras RT, Streppel MT, Draijer R, Zock PL. Flow-mediated dilation and cardiovascular risk prediction: a systematic review with meta-analysis. *International journal of cardiology*. 2013; 168:344–351. [PubMed: 23041097].

[121] Lavi S, Bae JH, Rihal CS, Prasad A, Barsness GW, Lennon RJ, Holmes DR Jr, Lerman A. Segmental coronary endothelial dysfunction in patients with minimal atherosclerosis is associated with necrotic core plaques. *Heart* (British Cardiac Society). 2009; 95:1525–1530. [PubMed: 19497916].

[122] Lerman A, Edwards BS, Hallett JW, Heublein DM, Sandberg SM, Burnett JC Jr. Circulating and tissue endothelin immunoreactivity in advanced atherosclerosis. *The New England journal of medicine*. 1991; 325:997–1001. [PubMed: 1886637].

[123] Stone GW, Maehara A, Lansky AJ, de Bruyne B, Cristea E, Mintz GS, Mehran R, McPherson J, Farhat N, Marso SP, Parise H, Templin B, White R, Zhang Z, Serruys PW. A prospective natural-history study of coronary atherosclerosis. *The New England journal of medicine*. 2011; 364:226–235. [PubMed: 21247313].

[124] Hambrecht R, Wolf A, Gielen S, Linke A, Hofer J, Erbs S, Schoene N, Schuler G. Effect of exercise on coronary endothelial function in patients with coronary artery disease. *The New England journal of medicine*. 2000; 342:454–460. [PubMed: 10675425].

[125] Clarkson P, Montgomery HE, Mullen MJ, Donald AE, Powe AJ, Bull T, Jubb M, World M, Deanfield JE. Exercise training enhances endothelial function in young men. *Journal of the American College of Cardiology*. 1999; 33:1379–1385. [PubMed: 10193742].

[126] Hambrecht R, Fiehn E, Weigl C, Gielen S, Hamann C, Kaiser R, Yu J, Adams V, Niebauer J, Schuler G. Regular physical exercise corrects endothelial dysfunction and improves exercise capacity in patients with chronic heart failure. *Circulation*. 1998; 98:2709–2715. [PubMed: 9851957].

[127] Dod HS, Bhardwaj R, Sajja V, Weidner G, Hobbs GR, Konat GW, Manivannan S, Gharib W, Warden BE, Nanda NC, Beto RJ, Ornish D, Jain AC. Effect of intensive lifestyle changes on endothelial function and on inflammatory markers of atherosclerosis. *The American journal of cardiology*. 2010; 105:362–367. [PubMed: 20102949].

[128] Meyer AA, Kundt G, Lenschow U, Schuff-Werner P, Kienast W. Improvement of early vascular changes and cardiovascular risk factors in obese children after a six-month exercise program. *Journal of the American College of Cardiology*. 2006; 48:1865–1870. [PubMed: 17084264].

[129] Shechter M, Beigel R, Freimark D, Matetzky S, Feinberg MS. Short-term sibutramine therapy is associated with weight loss and improved endothelial function in obese patients with coronary artery disease. *The American journal of cardiology*. 2006; 97:1650–1653. [PubMed: 16728231].

[130] Sturm W, Tschoner A, Engl J, Kaser S, Laimer M, Ciardi C, Klaus A, Weiss H, Sandhofer A, Patsch JR, Ebenbichler CF. Effect of bariatric surgery on both functional and structural measures of premature atherosclerosis. *European heart journal*. 2009; 30:2038–2043. [PubMed: 19502233].

[131] Gokce N, Vita JA, McDonnell M, Forse AR, Istfan N, Stoeckl M, Lipinska I, Keaney JF Jr, Apovian CM. Effect of medical and surgical weight loss on endothelial vasomotor function in obese patients. *The American journal of cardiology*. 2005; 95:266–268. [PubMed: 15642566].

[132] Corti R, Flammer AJ, Hollenberg NK, Luscher TF. Cocoa and cardiovascular health. *Circulation*. 2009; 119:1433–1441. [PubMed: 19289648].

[133] Flammer AJ, Hermann F, Sudano I, Spieker L, Hermann M, Cooper KA, Serafini M, Luscher TF, Ruschitzka F, Noll G, Corti R. Dark chocolate improves coronary vasomotion and reduces platelet reactivity. *Circulation*. 2007; 116:2376–2382. [PubMed: 17984375].

[134] Sudano I, Spieker LE, Hermann F, Flammer A, Corti R, Noll G, Luscher TF. Protection of endothelial function: targets for nutritional and pharmacological interventions. *J Cardiovasc Pharmacol.* 2006; 47(Suppl 2):S136–150. discussion S172-136. [PubMed: 16794451].

[135] Reriani MK, Dunlay SM, Gupta B, West CP, Rihal CS, Lerman LO, Lerman A. Effects of statins on coronary and peripheral endothelial function in humans: a systematic review and metaanalysis of randomized controlled trials. *Eur J Cardiovasc Prev Rehabil.* 2011.

[136] Anderson TJ, Meredith IT, Yeung AC, Frei B, Selwyn AP, Ganz P. The effect of cholesterollowering and antioxidant therapy on endothelium-dependent coronary vasomotion. *The New England journal of medicine.* 1995; 332:488–493. [PubMed: 7830729].

[137] Treasure CB, Klein JL, Weintraub WS, Talley JD, Stillabower ME, Kosinski AS, Zhang J, Boccuzzi SJ, Cedarholm JC, Alexander RW. Beneficial effects of cholesterol-lowering therapy on the coronary endothelium in patients with coronary artery disease. *The New England journal of medicine.* 1995; 332:481–487. [PubMed: 7830728].

[138] Bonetti PO, Lerman LO, Napoli C, Lerman A. Statin effects beyond lipid lowering--are they clinically relevant? *European heart journal.* 2003; 24:225–248. [PubMed: 12590901].

[139] Lüscher TF, Vanhoutte PM, Raij L. Antihypertensive treatment normalizes decreased endothelium-dependent relaxations in rats with salt-induced hypertension. *Hypertension.* 1987; 9 (Suppl III):193–197.

[140] Taddei S, Virdis A, Ghiadoni L, Sudano I, Salvetti A. Effects of antihypertensive drugs on endothelial dysfunction: clinical implications. *Drugs.* 2002; 62:265–284. [PubMed: 11817973]

[141] Mancini GB, Henry GC, Macaya C, O'Neill BJ, Pucillo AL, Carere RG, Wargovich TJ, Mudra H, Luscher TF, Klibaner MI, Haber HE, Uprichard AC, Pepine CJ, Pitt B. Angiotensinconverting enzyme inhibition with quinapril improves endothelial vasomotor

dysfunction in patients with coronary artery disease. The TREND (Trial on Reversing ENdothelial Dysfunction) Study. *Circulation.* 1996; 94:258–265. [PubMed: 8759064].

[142] Chen JW, Hsu NW, Wu TC, Lin SJ, Chang MS. Long-term angiotensin-converting enzyme inhibition reduces plasma asymmetric dimethylarginine and improves endothelial nitric oxide bioavailability and coronary microvascular function in patients with syndrome X. *The American journal of cardiology*. 2002; 90:974–982. [PubMed: 12398965].

[143] Taddei S, Virdis A, Ghiadoni L, Mattei P, Salvetti A. Effects of angiotensin converting enzyme inhibition on endothelium-dependent vasodilatation in essential hypertensive patients. *J Hypertens*. 1998; 16:447–456. [PubMed: 9797190].

[144] Creager MA, Roddy M-A, Coleman SM, Dzau VJ. The effect of ACE inhibition on endotheliumdependent vasodilation in hypertension. *J Vasc Res*. 1992; 29:97.

[145] Flammer AJ, Hermann F, Wiesli P, Schwegler B, Chenevard R, Hurlimann D, Sudano I, Gay S, Neidhart M, Riesen W, Ruschitzka F, Luscher TF, Noll G, Lehmann R. Effect of losartan, compared with atenolol, on endothelial function and oxidative stress in patients with type 2 diabetes and hypertension. *J Hypertens*. 2007; 25:785–791. [PubMed: 17351370].

[146] Effect of nifedipine and cerivastatin on coronary endothelial function in patients with coronary artery disease: the ENCORE I Study (Evaluation of Nifedipine and Cerivastatin on Recovery of coronary Endothelial function). *Circulation.* 2003; 107:422–428. [PubMed: 12551866].

[147] Taddei S, Virdis A, Ghiadoni L, Uleri S, Magagna A, Salvetti A. Lacidipine restores endothelium-dependent vasodilation in essential hypertensive patients. *Hypertension.* 1997; 30:1606–1612. [PubMed: 9403590].

[148] Tang EH, Vanhoutte PM. Endothelial dysfunction: a strategic target in the treatment of hypertension? *Pflugers Arch.* 459:995–1004. [PubMed: 20127126].

[149] Luscher TF, Pieper M, Tendera M, Vrolix M, Rutsch W, van den Branden F, Gil R, Bischoff KO, Haude M, Fischer D, Meinertz T, Munzel T. A randomized placebo-controlled study on the effect of nifedipine on coronary endothelial function and plaque formation in patients with coronary artery disease: the ENCORE II study. *European heart journal.* 2009; 30:1590–1597. [PubMed: 19474053].

[150] Prisant LM. Nebivolol: pharmacologic profile of an ultraselective, vasodilatory beta1-blocker. *J Clin Pharmacol.* 2008; 48:225–239. [PubMed: 18083889].

[151] Taddei S, Virdis A, Ghiadoni L, Magagna A, Salvetti A. Vitamin C improves endotheliumdependent vasodilation by restoring nitric oxide activity in essential hypertension. *Circulation.* 1998; 97:2222–2229. [PubMed: 9631871]

[152] Kinlay S, Behrendt D, Fang JC, Delagrange D, Morrow J, Witztum JL, Rifai N, Selwyn AP, Creager MA, Ganz P. Long-term effect of combined vitamins E and C on coronary and peripheral endothelial function. *Journal of the American College of Cardiology.* 2004; 43:629– 634. [PubMed: 14975474].

[153] Sherman DL, Keaney JF Jr, Biegelsen ES, Duffy SJ, Coffman JD, Vita JA. Pharmacological concentrations of ascorbic acid are required for the beneficial effect on endothelial vasomotor function in hypertension. *Hypertension.* 2000; 35:936–941. [PubMed: 10775565]

[154] Versari D, Daghini E, Rodriguez-Porcel M, Sattler K, Galili O, Pilarczyk K, Napoli C, Lerman LO, Lerman A. Chronic antioxidant supplementation impairs coronary endothelial function and myocardial perfusion in normal pigs. *Hypertension.* 2006; 47:475–481. [PubMed: 16446399].

[155] Ganz P, Hsue PY. Individualized approach to the management of coronary heart disease: identifying the nonresponders before it is too late. *Journal of the American College of Cardiology.* 2009; 53:331–333. [PubMed: 19161881].

[156] Elbaz M, Carrie D, Baudeux JL, et al. High frequency of endothelial vasomotor dysfunction after acute coronary syndromes in non-culprit and angiographically normal coronary arteries: a reversible phenomenon. *Atherosclerosis.* 2005; 181:311–319. [PubMed: 16039285].

[157] Greenland P, Alpert JS, Beller GA, Benjamin EJ, Budoff MJ, Fayad ZA, Foster E, Hlatky MA, Hodgson JM, Kushner FG, Lauer MS, Shaw LJ, Smith SC Jr, Taylor AJ, Weintraub WS, Wenger NK, Jacobs AK. 2010 ACCF/AHA guideline for assessment of cardiovascular risk in asymptomatic adults: a report of the American College of Cardiology Foundation/American Heart Association Task Force on Practice Guidelines. *Circulation.* 2010; 122:e584–636. [PubMed: 21098428].

[158] Brindle P, Emberson J, Lampe F, Walker M, Whincup P, Fahey T, Ebrahim S. Predictive accuracy of the Framingham coronary risk score in British men: prospective cohort study. *BMJ.* 2003; 327:1267. [PubMed: 14644971].

In: A Closer Look at Cardiovascular … ISBN: 978-1-53613-939-6
Editor: Faris van Kilsdonk

Chapter 3

CARDIOVASCULAR RISK FACTORS AND SENSORINEURAL HEARING LOSS

V. Corazzi, C. Bianchini, C. Aimoni and A. Ciorba**[*]**
ENT & Audiology Department, University Hospital of Ferrara, Ferrara, Italy

ABSTRACT

The inner ear may be impaired by vascular affections since it is supplied by a terminal blood flow and has a sustained metabolic activity [1]. It has been reported that the function of labyrinthine vessels can be influenced by several local factors such as perivascular sympathetic innervation, arterial systemic blood pressure and labyrinth liquids pressure ratio, antidiuretic hormone receptors, endothelial dysfunction and ionic transport mechanisms [2].

A possible link between microvascular inner ear disease and sudden sensorineural hearing loss (SSNHL) has been proposed: a sudden labyrinth oxygen lack may be responsible for acute inner ear damage, involving hair cells and then affecting hearing or vestibular function [3]. Moreover, a primary autonomic vascular dysregulation has been related to acute cochlear damage [2]. Many Authors have investigated the

[*] Corresponding Author Email: andrea.ciorba@unife.it.

possible involvement of cardiovascular risk factors (i.e., hypertension, diabetes mellitus, hypercholesterolemia, hyperhomocysteinemia) in the pathogenesis of sudden sensorineural hearing loss [4]. Furthermore, microcirculation defects, frequently associated to atherosclerosis, have been reported to play a major role in the onset of acute cochlear damage [5].

The aim of this chapter is to review the relationship between cardiovascular risk factors, systemic circulatory diseases and inner ear disorders, particularly focusing on the involvement of cardiovascular factors in the pathogenesis of SSNHL.

Keywords: sensorineural hearing loss, sudden sensorineural hearing loss, cardiovascular risk factors, hypertension, diabetes mellitus, smoking

INTRODUCTION

The inner ear is a sensorial organ characterized by neuroepithelial cells with a high oxygen-dependent metabolism. Its vascularization is provided by a terminal circulation: the labyrinthine artery is a branch of the anterior inferior cerebellar artery (rarely of the basilar artery directly) and it is the only vessel responsible for the inner ear blood supply [1]. This anatomic and functional configuration (in particular, the absence of collateral vessels and the sustained metabolic activity of the inner ear cells) represents the main reason for the high sensitivity of the inner ear to vascular accidents [1]. There are three terminal branches originating from the labyrinthine artery: (1) the anterior vestibular, (2) the vestibulocochlear and (3) the main cochlear artery, which supply different parts of the inner ear (vestibular and cochlear partitions) [1]. Towards the terminal extremity of these vessels, the arteries decrease in size and lose their muscular layers, therefore increasing their predisposition to peripheral vasomotion disorders [6]. This vascular subdivision represents the anatomical explanation for the different clinical features (matching hearing loss and vertigo) resulting from vascular accidents, such as localized ischemic events [7]. Therefore, alteration of platelet aggregation, red cells deformability, haematocrit and plasmatic viscosity (as described in several conditions such as leukaemia, leucocytosis, polycythaemia, sickle-cell anaemia, cryoglobulinemia, macroglobulinemia) may have implications also on inner ear function [8].

There are several local factors influencing the inner ear perfusion, such as perivascular sympathetic innervation, arterial systemic blood pressure or labyrinthic liquids pressure ratio [2]. The labyrinthic blood flow is also regulated by blood labyrinthine barrier, pericytes, smooth muscle cells and fibrocytes; endothelial dysfunction and alterations of ionic transport could represent another mechanism of cochlear injury, as well [9].

Concerning the autonomic nervous system control on local inner ear perfusion [10, 11], the function of distal arterioles has been reported to affect directly the number of perfused capillaries and the partition of local blood distribution. In particular, many studies have focused on stria vascularis capillaries and on their capacity to interact with different signals, such as iron ions and nitric oxide in presence of an acoustic stimulus, then determining an increase of local blood flow [12].

Alterations of the intracranial venous circulation have been related to the pathogenesis of inner ear disorders, in consideration of the delicate balance existing between intracranial and labyrinthic fluids pressure; it has been reported that a variation of venous pressure may interfere with inner ear homeostasis [13, 14, 15].

Sensorineural Hearing Loss and Cardiovascular Risk Factors

The inner ear may be damaged by hemodynamic or metabolic events in case of systemic diseases, such as cardiovascular, renal, inflammatory, autoimmune and/or metabolic disorders [16]. Hearing loss has been related to cardiovascular risk factors (such as male gender, hypertension, dyslipidaemia, obesity, lack of physical activity, diabetes mellitus, atherosclerosis, smoking) and also, in the Framingham Heart Study, to cardiovascular events, such as cerebrovascular and coronary artery disease [16, 17, 18]. In addition, other cardiovascular risk factors, such as body mass index, waist circumference and socioeconomic status, have been found to be linked to the incidence of hearing loss in longitudinal studies [19, 20, 21].

Obesity has been considered to cause inner ear cells injury through ischaemic damage and oxidative stress, the same mechanisms through which tobacco, potentially, could act as risk factor for hearing loss [21].

High systolic blood pressure (more than the diastolic) was found to have a positive correlation with hearing loss in frequencies above 500Hz [22].

Increased blood sugar levels may damage the vascular endothelial walls. Moreover, an increased prevalence of hearing loss has been reported in patients with an impaired glucose control [23]. In 2006 Fukushima demonstrated a condition of angiopathy and degeneration of outer hair cells and of stria vascularis examining temporal bones of diabetic patients [24].

Elevated lipid blood levels (low-density lipoproteins in particular) have been linked to microvascular damage [25], nonetheless a direct association between blood lipids and hearing loss has not been demonstrated yet [26].

Recently, the relationship between hearing loss and levels of serum C-reactive protein (CRP), another cardiovascular risk marker, has been investigated; Nash [27] found an increased 10-year risk of hearing loss in case of high levels of CRP [26], but further confirms are necessary.

Subclinical atherosclerosis has been related to an increased incidence of hearing loss in a large cohort study (1984 middle-aged patients - increased risk of about 15%) [28]. Atherosclerotic plaques may affect inner ear perfusion due to a decreased availability of oxygen and nutrients to the cochlea [22]. In 1978, Makishima found a positive association between (i) the narrowing of the internal auditory artery, (ii) stria vascularis atrophy, and (iii) hearing loss, suggesting that a spiral ganglion atrophy could result from a chronic reduction of cochlear blood flow caused by atherosclerosis [29]. However, the precise role of atherosclerosis, as a risk factor for hearing impairment, has not been completely understood [17], since systemic atherosclerosis may also coexist with a normal hearing function [30].

Presbycusis is among the most frequent sensorial deficit in elderly and its prevalence increases with age, as much as cardiovascular diseases [31]. Since cardiovascular risk factors are generally more frequent in the elderly, it could be difficult to distinguish the effects of cardiovascular diseases on inner ear function, from those related to (i) ageing, (ii) occupational or environmental noise exposure, or (iii) use of ototoxic drugs[17, 32].

The interaction between presbycusis and diabetes mellitus has been investigated [33]. Frisina studied a population of aged diabetic patients compared to age-matched healthy control patients, performing both peripheral and central auditory tests [33]: the Author evidenced significant differences between the two groups in both auditory categories tests with poorer performances in the diabetics group, highlighting that hyperglycemia may damage not only the inner ear cells, but also the central nervous system.

SUDDEN SENSORINEURAL HEARING LOSS AND CARDIOVASCULAR RISK FACTORS

To date, the pathogenesis of idiopathic sudden sensorineural hearing loss (SSNHL) remains unclear. Among the different etiopathogenetic hypotheses, the vascular theory is one of the most investigated [6, 34]. Several Authors evaluated the existence of a link between cardiovascular factors and the onset of sudden hearing loss [7, 8, 35]. Marcucci [8] and Capaccio [36] found an increased concentration of cholesterol, fibrinogen and homocysteine as cardiovascular risk factors in patients affected by SSNHL. In addition, several inherited and acquired cardiovascular risk factors have been found to increase the risk of hearing impairment development: Ballesteros [35] found a higher prevalence of the 807T thrombophilic polymorphism of platelet glycoprotein Ia/IIa in patients affected by idiopathic SSNHL compared to healthy control patients and assessed a poorer hearing recovery rate in patients homozygous for this polymorphism.

Aimoni et al. [4] evidenced hypercholesterolemia and diabetes mellitus (particularly associated with insulin therapy) to be significantly more frequent in patients affected by SSNHL and, later, Chang [25] found the same two issues to be independent risk factors for SSNHL, even if some conflicting data exist [37].

Mosnier [7] did not find any significant difference in the prevalence of cardiovascular risk factors (such as total lipids, diabetes mellitus, and smoking) among patients with SSNHL and the healthy controls, whereas reported that cardiovascular accidents (including myocardial infarction, stroke, transient ischemic attack) were significantly more prevalent in patients with SSNHL.

In a case-control study, Ciccone et al. [38] found a significant lower flow-mediated dilation of the brachial artery and significant higher total cholesterol and low density lipoprotein cholesterol blood levels in patients affected by SSNHL compared to the healthy control group, suggesting a possible correlation between idiopathic SSNHL and vascular endothelial disorder. Previously, Balletshofer [39] found that 5 out of 6 patients affected by idiopathic SSNHL showed endothelial dysfunction, supporting an involvement of microcirculation disorders in the pathogenesis of hearing impairment.

In a large cohort-control study, a higher risk of stroke (1.64 rate) has been estimated in patients with idiopathic SSNHL [40].

Keller [41] found an association between acute myocardial infarction and previous onset of SSNHL; Lin [42] defined SSNHL as a possible independent risk factor for myocardial infarction, in particular for patients aged $\geq$ 50 years. These observations may allow considering SSNHL as a possible predictor of major cardiovascular accidents [40, 41, 42].

In 2015, Pirodda speculated a possible involvement of a primary autonomic vascular dysregulation in the acute cochlear damage [43]. The primary vascular dysregulation syndrome, a condition of inappropriate vasoconstriction and vasodilatations of arteries, veins and capillaries, has been previously associated to several ophthalmological diseases [44]. In this syndrome low blood pressure, minor resistance to psychological stress, major sensitivity to pain, autonomic imbalance, migraine are often present [44] and have been linked also to the onset of a labyrinthine acute impairment [43]. Schulz and co-workers showed an altered autonomic regulation in patients affected by idiopathic SSNHL, particularly demonstrating modifications in their blood pressure regulation, in comparison to normal hearing patients [45, 46, 47]. Hultcrantz and collaborators [10] supposed that in case of reduced cochlear blood flow (i.e., in case of hypotension), cochlear circulation could depend on sympathetic tone.

The involvement of cardiovascular risk factors in the pathogenesis of idiopathic SSNHL seems to be plausible, but remains a hypothesis to date. The role of cardiovascular risk factors in hearing threshold recovery after a SSNHL is also unclear [48].

CONCLUSION

Micro-vascular defects can damage the inner ear, since it is a sensory-neural organ with a sustained metabolic activity, supplied by a terminal blood flow [1]. Many Authors have investigated the role of cardiovascular risk factors in the pathogenesis of hearing loss and, in particular, of idiopathic SSNHL [16-30, 34]. Even if, to date, clear evidences do not support the vascular etiopathogenetic hypothesis, it is possible to consider hearing disorders as a potential sign of circulatory instability [2, 21]. In this regard, there are also evidences supporting links between SSNHL and major cardiovascular diseases such as stroke [40, 41, 42]; a careful evaluation of cardiovascular risk factors should be recommended among these patients [21, 49].

For these reasons, in case of hearing impairment, Audiologist and Otolaryngologist should (i) investigate patients cardiovascular history, (ii) refer for blood tests, electrocardiogram and supra-aortic trunks ultrasound, (iii) possibly refer to a cardiologist for further diagnostic investigation and (iv) encourage patients to reduce modifiable cardiovascular risk factors.

REFERENCES

[1] Mudry, A.; Tange, R. A. The vascularization of the human cochlea its historical background. *Acta Oto-Laryngologica*, 2009; 129(Suppl. 561):3-16.

[2] Pirodda, A.; Cicero, A. F.; Brandolini, C.; Borghi, C. Inner ear symptoms: can we use them to approach cardiovascular diseases? *Intern. Emerg. Med.,* 2014; 9(8):825-7.

[3] Gyo, K. Experimental study of transient cochlear ischemia as a cause of sudden deafness. *World J. Otorhinolaryngol*., 2013; 3:1-15.

[4] Aimoni, C.; Bianchini, C.; Borin, M.; Ciorba, A.; Fellin, R.; Martini, A.; Scanelli, G.; Volpato, S. Diabetes, Cardiovascular Risk Factors and Idiopathic Sudden Sensorineural Hearing Loss: A Case-Control Study. *Audiol. Neurotol*., 2010; 15:111-115.

[5] Rajati, M.; Azarpajooh, M. R.; Mouhebati, M.; Nasrollahi, M.; Salehi, M.; Khadivi, E.; Nourizadeh, N.; Hashemi, F.; Bakhshaee, M. Is Sudden Hearing Loss Associated with Atherosclerosis? *Iran J. Otorhinolaryngol.,* 2016;28(86):189-95.

[6] Schuknecht, H. F.; Benitez, J.; Beekhuis, J.; Igarashi, M.; Singleton, G.; Ruedi, L. The pathology of sudden deafness. *Laryngoscope,* 1962; 72:1142-57.

[7] Mosnier, I.; Stepanian, A.; Baron, G.; Bodenez, C.; Robier, A.; Meyer, B.; Fraysse, B.; Bertholon, P.; Defay, F.; Ameziane, N.; Ferrary, E.; Sterkers, O.; de Prost, D. Cardiovascular and thromboembolic risk factors in idiopathic sudden sensorineural hearing loss: a case-control study. *Audiol. Neurootol.,* 2011; 16(1): 55-66.

[8] Marcucci, R.; Alessandrello Liotta, A.; Cellai, A. P.; Rogolino, A.; Berloco, P.; Leprini, E., Pagnini, P.; Abbate, R.; Prisco, D.; Cardiovascular and thrombophilic risk factors for idiopathic sudden sensorineural hearing loss. *J. Thromb. Haemost.,* 2005; 3:929-934.

[9] Shi, X. Physiopathology of the Cochlear Microcirculation. *Hear. Res.,* 2001; 282(1–2):10–24.

[10] Hultcrantz, E.; Linder, J.; Angelborg, C. Sympathetic effects on cochlear blood flow at different blood pressure levels. *INSERM,* 1977; 68:71Y8.

[11] Seidman, M. D.; Quirk, W. S.; Shirwany, N. A. Mechanisms of alterations in the microcirculation of the cochlea. *Ann. NY Acad. Sci.,* 1999; 884:226–32.

[12] Dai, M.; Shi, X. Fibro-vascular coupling in the control of cochlear blood flow. *PLoS. One.,* 2011; 6(6):e20652.

[13] Chiarella, G.; Bono, F.; Cassandro, C.; Lopolito, M.; Quattrone, A.; Cassandro, E. Bilateral transverse sinus stenosis in patients with tinnitus. *Acta. Otorhinolaryngol. Ital.,* 2012; 32(4):238-43.

[14] Dietz, R. R.; Davis, W. L.; Harnsberger, H. R.; Jacobs, J. M.; Blatter, D. D. MR imaging and MR angiography in the evaluation of pulsatile tinnitus. *AJNR*, 1994; 15:879-889.

[15] Koenigsberg, R. A. Spontaneous pulsatile tinnitus secondary to a dural malformation not visualized by magnetic resonance angiography. *Clinical imaging,* 1996; 20:95-98.

[16] Pirodda, A.; Brandolini, C.; Ferri, G. G.; Modugno, G. C.; Degli Esposti, D.; Borghi, C. Inner ear dysfunction of uncertain origin: a multidisciplinary approach could give something more. *Med. Hypotheses,* 2009; 72:188–189.

[17] Oron, Y.; Elgart, K.; Marom, T.; Roth, Y. Cardiovascular risk factors as causes for hearing impairment. *Audiol. Neurotol.,* 2014; 19: 256-60.

[18] Gates, G. A.; Cobb, J. L.; D'Agostino, R. B.; Wolf, P. A. The relation of hearing in the elderly to the presence of cardiovascular disease and cardiovascular risk factors. *Arch. Otolaryngol. Head Neck Surg.,* 1993; 119(2):156-161.

[19] Curhan, S. G.; Eavey, R.; Wang, M.; Stampfer, M. J.; Curhan, G. C. Body mass index, waist circumference, physical activity, and risk of hearing loss in women. *Am. J. Med.,* 2013; 126(12):1142.e1-1142.e8.

[20] Linssen, A. M.; van Boxtel, M. P.; Joore, M. A.; Anteunis, L. J. Predictors of hearing acuity: cross-sectional and longitudinal analysis. *J. Gerontol. A. Biol. Sci. Med. Sci.,* 2014; 69(6):759-765.

[21] Tan, H. E.; Lan, N. S. R.; Knuiman, M. W.; Divitini, M. L.; Swanepoel, D. W.; Hunter, M.; Brennan-Jones, C. G.; Hung, J.; Eikelboom, R. H.; Santa Maria, P. L. Associations between cardiovascular disease and its risk factors with hearing loss-A cross-sectional analysis. *Clin. Otolaryngol.,* 2018; 43(1):172-181.

[22] Brant, L. J.; Gordon-Salant, S.; Pearson, J. D.; Klein, L. L.; Morrell, C. H.; Metter, E. J.; Fozard, J. L. Risk factors related to age-associated hearing loss in the speech frequencies. *J. Am. Acad. Audiol.,* 1996; 7: 152-160.

[23] Oiticica, J.; Bittar, S. Metabolic disorders prevalence in sudden deafness. *Clinics,* 2010; 65:1149-1153.

[24] Fukushima, H.; Cureoglu, S.; Schachern, P. A.; Paparella, M. M.; Harada, T.; Oktay, M. F. Effects of type 2 diabetes mellitus on cochlear structure in humans. *Arch. Otolaryngol. Head Neck. Surg.,* 2006; 132: 934-938.

[25] Chang, S. L.; Hsieh, C. C.; Tseng, K. S.; Weng, S. F.; Lyn, Y. S. Hypercholesterolemia is correlated with an increased risk of idiopathic sudden sensorineural hearing loss: a historical prospective cohort study. *Ear. Hear.,* 2014; 35:256-261.

[26] Simpson, A. N.; Matthews, L. J.; Dubno, J. R. Lipid and C-reactive protein levels as risk factors for hearing loss in older adults. *Otolaryngol. Head Neck Surg.,* 2013; 148(4):664-70.

[27] Nash, S. D.; Cruickshanks, K. J.; Klein, R.; Klein, B. E.; Nieto, F. J.; Chappell, R.; Schubert, C. R.; Tsai, M. Y. Long-term variability of inflammatory markers and associated factors in a population-based cohort. *J. Am. Geriatr. Soc.,* 2013; 61(8):1269-1276.

[28] Fischer, M. E.; Schubert, C. R.; Nondahl, D. M.; Dalton, D. S.; Huang, G. H.; Keating, B. J.; Klein, B. E.; Klein, R.; Tweed, T. S. Cruickshanks KJ10. Subclinical atherosclerosis and increased risk of hearing impairment. *Atherosclerosis,* 2015; 238(2):344-9.

[29] Makishima, K. Arteriolar sclerosis as a cause of presbycusis. *Otolaryngology,* 1978; 86:322-326.

[30] Pirodda, A.; Brandolini, C.; Borghi, C. The influence of systemic circulation on hearing: The reliability of a different impact of

microcirculatory defects and atherosclerosis. *Med. Hypotheses.,* 2016; 91:6-8.

[31] Benjamin, E. J.; Blaha, M. J.; Chiuve, S. E.; Cushman, M.; Das, S. R.; Deo, R.; de Ferranti, S. D.; Floyd, J.; Fornage, M.; Gillespie, C.; Isasi, C. R.; Jiménez, M. C.; Jordan, L. C.; Judd, S. E.; Lackland, D.; Lichtman, J. H.; Lisabeth, L.; Liu, S.; Longenecker, C. T.; Mackey, R. H.; Matsushita, K.; Mozaffarian, D.; Mussolino, M. E.; Nasir, K.; Neumar, R. W.; Palaniappan, L.; Pandey, D. K.; Thiagarajan, R. R.; Reeves, M. J.; Ritchey, M.; Rodriguez, C. J.; Roth, G. A.; Rosamond, W. D.; Sasson, C.; Towfighi, A.; Tsao, C. W.; Turner, M. B.; Virani, S. S.; Voeks, J. H.; Willey, J. Z.; Wilkins, J. T., Wu, J. H., Alger, H. M.; Wong, S. S.; Muntner, P.; American Heart Association Statistics Committee and Stroke Statistics Subcommittee. Heart Disease and Stroke Statistics-2017 Update: A Report from the American Heart Association. *Circulation,* 2017; 135(10):e146-e603.

[32] Cruickshanks, K. J.; Nondahl, D. M.; Dalton, D. S.; Fischer, M. E.; Klein, B. E.; Klein, R.; Nieto, F. J.; Schubert, C. R.; Tweed, T. S. Smoking, central adiposity, and poor glycemic control increase risk of hearing impairment. *J. Am. Geriatr. Soc.,* 2015; 63(5):918-24.

[33] Frisina, S. T.; Mapes, F.; Kim, S.; Frisina, D. R.; Frisina, R. D. Characterization of hearing loss in aged type II diabetics. *Hear. Res.,* 2006; 211(1-2):103-13.

[34] Trune, D. R.; Nguyen-Huynh, A. Vascular Pathophysiology in Hearing Disorders. *Semin. Hear.,* 2012; 33(3):242-250.

[35] Ballesteros, F.; Alobid, I.; Tassies, D.; Reverter, J. C.; Scharf, R. E.; Guilemany, J. M.; Bernal-Sprekelsen, M. Is there an overlap between sudden neurosensorial hearing loss and cardiovascular risk factors? *Audiol. Neurootol.,* 2009; 14:139-145.

[36] Capaccio, P.; Ottaviani, F.; Cuccarini, V.; Bottero, A.; Schindler, A.; Cessana, B. M.; Censuales, S.; Pignataro, L. Genetic and acquired prothrombotic risk factors and sudden hearing loss. *Laryngoscope,* 2007; 117: 547–551.

[37] Rudack, C.; Langer, C.; Stoll, W.; Rust, S.; Walter, M. Vascular risk factors in sudden hearing loss. *Thromb. Haemost.,* 2006; 95(3): 454-61.

[38] Ciccone, M. M.; Cortese, F.; Pinto, M.; Di Teo, C.; Fornarelli, F.; Gesualdo, M.; Mezzina, A.; Sabatelli, E.; Scicchitano, P.; Quaranta, N. Endothelial function and cardiovascular risk in patients with Idiopathic Sudden Sensorineural Hearing Loss. *Atherosclerosis,* 2012; 225(2):511-6.

[39] Balletshofer, B. M.; Stock, J.; Rittig, K.; Lehn-Stefan, A.; Braun, N.; Burkart, F.; Plontke, S.; Klingel, R.; Häring, H. U. Acute effect of rheopheresis on peripheral endothelial dysfunction in patients suffering from sudden hearing loss. *Ther. Apher. Dial.,* 2005; 9(5): 385-90.

[40] Lin, H. C.; Chao, P. Z.; Lee, H. C. Sudden sensorineural hearing loss increases the risk of stroke: a 5-year follow-up study. *Stroke,* 2008; 39:2744Y8.

[41] Keller, J. J.; Wu, C. S.; Kang, J. H.; Lin, H. C. Association of acute myocardial infarction with sudden sensorineural hearing loss: a population-based case-control study. *Audiol. Neurootol.,* 2013; 18(1): 3-8.

[42] Lin, C.; Lin, S. W.; Lin, Y. S.; Weng, S. F., Lee, T. M. Sudden sensorineural hearing loss is correlated with an increased risk of acute myocardial infarction: a population-based cohort study. *Laryngoscope,* 2013; 123(9):2254-8.

[43] Pirodda, A.; Brandolini, C.; Cassandro, E.; Borghi, C. Primary vascular dysregulation syndrome: Possible implications for inner ear acute diseases? *Med. Hypotheses.,* 2015; 85(5):586-7.

[44] Flammer, J.; Konieczka, K.; Flammer, A. J. The primary vascular dysregulation syndrome: implications for eye diseases. *EPMA J.,* 2013; 4(1):14.

[45] Schulz, S.; Witt, K.; Fischer, C.; Bär, K. J.; Ritter, J.; Guntinas-Lichius, O.; Voss, A. Altered cardiovascular coupling in patients with sudden sensorineural hearing loss in comparison to healthy

subjects. *Conf. Proc. IEEE. Eng. Med. Biol. Soc.,* 2013; 2013: 3933Y6.

[46] Schulz, S.; Ritter, J.; Oertel, K.; Witt, K.; Bär, K. J.; Guntinas-Lichius, O., Voss, A. Quantification of autonomic regulation in patients with sudden sensorineural hearing loss. *Auton. Neurosci.,* 2013; 178:9Y14.

[47] Schulz, S., Ritter, J.; Oertel, K.; Witt, K.; Bär, K. J.; Guntinas-Lichius, O.; Voss, A. Altered autonomic regulation as a cardiovascular risk marker for patients with sudden sensorineural hearing loss. *Otol. Neurotol.,* 2014; 35(10):1720-9.

[48] Ciorba, A.; Hatzopoulos, S.; Bianchini, C.; Iannini, V.; Rosignoli, M.; Skarzynski, H.; Aimoni, C. Idiopathic sudden sensorineural hearing loss: cardiovascular risk factors do not influence hearing threshold recovery. *Acta. Otorhinolaryngol. Ital.,* 2015; 35(2):103-9.

[49] Haremza, C.; Klopp-Dutote, N.; Strunski, V.; Page, C. Evaluation of cardiovascular risks and recovery of idiopathic sudden sensorineural hearing loss in hospitalised patients: comparison between complete and partial sudden sensorineural hearing loss. *J. Laryngol. Otol.,* 2017; 131(10):919-924.

In: A Closer Look at Cardiovascular … ISBN: 978-1-53613-939-6
Editor: Faris van Kilsdonk

Chapter 4

IMPROVEMENT OF CARDIOVASCULAR RISK FACTORS AFTER BARIATRIC SURGERY

***Jaime Ruiz-Tovar*[1] *and Carolina Llavero*[2]**
[1]Department of Surgery. Centro de Excelencia para el Estudio y Tratamiento de la Obesidad, Valladolid, Spain
[2]Department of Surgical Nursery. Hospital del Sureste. Madrid, Spain

ABSTRACT

Impaired glucose tolerance, hypertension, and dyslipidemia have been described as metabolic syndrome (MetS). MetS is associated with an increased cardiovascular risk. A close association between morbid obesity and MetS has been highlighted in several clinical studies. Disease risk increases with increasing body mass index (BMI). However, BMI can be misleading for certain body constitutions. Thus, other parameters have been proposed as predictors of cardiovascular risk. Among them, the adiposity, the Framingham Index and the Atherogenic Index (Triglycerids/HDL-c.).

Bariatric surgery has been shown to be effective in achieving and maintaining weight change and reducing obesity-related comorbidities. Malabsorptive procedures (biliopancreatic diversion and duodenal switch) have been associated with the greatest reduction of cardiovascular risk, associated with a greatest improvement in obesity-related comorbidities (diabetes mellitus, hypertension and dyslipidemia). On the other hand, the lowest improvement is obtained after restrictive procedures (Adjustable gastric banding (AGB). However, despite sleeve gastrectomy is also considered a restrictive procedure, the reported improvement of cardiovascular risk reduction is greater than after AGB, as a certain hormonal effect is also involved in this technique-

In this chapter we will review the current evidence of obesity-related comorbidities and cardiovascular risk factor index after different bariatric approaches.

INTRODUCTION

More than 2/3 of the U.S. population is overweight or obese. Obesity is on the rise and the incidence is increasing most rapidly in the morbidly obese population, i.e., those with BMIs exceeding 40 kg/m2. Epidemiological studies estimate the prevalence of morbid obesity around 0.5%, but this rate is probably underestimated, as many morbidly obese subjects are not under any medical control. Only surgery results in substantial, long-term weight loss for obese individuals. Therefore, the performance of bariatric procedure has increased exponentially in the last 2 decades; from less than 9,000 procedures in 1993 to a high of over 115,000 in 2004. It is estimated that 220,000 weight-loss surgeries were performed in 2008. Actually, the number of bariatric procedures performed is even higher [1].

Impaired glucose tolerance, hypertension, and dyslipidemia have been described as metabolic syndrome (MetS). MetS is associated with an increased cardiovascular risk. A close association between morbid obesity and MetS has been highlighted in several clinical studies. Disease risk increases with increasing body mass index (BMI) [2].

Bariatric surgery has been shown to be effective in achieving and maintaining weight change and reducing obesity-related comorbidities. Malabsorptive procedures (biliopancreatic diversion and duodenal switch) have been associated with the greatest reduction of cardiovascular risk, associated with a greatest improvement in obesity-related comorbidities (diabetes mellitus, hypertension and dyslipidemia). On the other hand, the lowest improvement is obtained after restrictive procedures (Adjustable gastric banding (AGB). Despite sleeve gastrectomy is also considered a restrictive procedure, the reported improvement of cardiovascular risk reduction is greater than after AGB. It has been hypothesized that a certain hormonal effect is also involved in this technique [3].

Disease risk increases with increasing body mass index (BMI). However, BMI can be misleading for certain body constitutions. Thus, other parameters have been proposed as predictors of cardiovascular risk. Among them, the adiposity, the Framingham Index and the Atherogenic Index (Triglycerids/HDL-c.) [2, 4].

Diabetes Mellitus

Bariatric surgical procedures are effective interventions for treating type 2 diabetes. Improvement in metabolic control is often evident within days to weeks following bariatric procedures, most likely reflecting an alteration in metabolism that is independent of weight loss [5].

Three randomized trials illustrate the efficacy of weight loss surgery versus medical therapy alone:

- Obese patients with uncontrolled type II diabetes, undergoing a RYGB or a SG plus medical therapy, were significantly more likely to achieve the main outcome of a glycated hemoglobin level of 6% or less at 12 months, compared with patients managed by intensive medical therapy alone (42% versus 37% versus 12%, respectively) [6].
- A randomized trial of 60 patients also found that obese diabetic patients undergoing a bariatric operation had better control than medical management alone. Obese patients (BMI ≥35) with a history of diabetes for five or more years and a glycated hemoglobin level ≥7%, undergoing a RYGB or biliopancreatic diversion (BPD), were significantly more likely to achieve the study endpoint of remission of diabetes at two years, compared

with patients managed by medical therapy alone (75% versus 95% versus 0%, respectively) [7].

- A randomized trial that included 120 patients demonstrated that a RYGB procedure was superior to intensive medical management alone in achieving the main outcome measure of a glycated hemoglobin level of less than 7%. (75% versus 32%) [8]. Results following RYGB operation are promising and several trials are in progress to evaluate the procedure for patients with BMI <35 and poorly controlled type 2 diabetes [9, 10]. Efficacious control of type 2 diabetes has also been demonstrated following a SG or an AGB.

In 2011, the American College of Surgeons Bariatric Surgery Center Network (ACSBSCN) found that the remission or improvement was for patients undergoing RYGB, SG, and AGB. In a prospective, longitudinal study, that included bariatric-specific data from more than 100 participating institutions and 28,616 obese diabetic patients, remission or improvement in diabetes at 12 months was achieved in 83% of patients undergoing a RYGB, 55% undergoing SG, and 44% undergoing an AGB [11]. This result has been corroborated by other studies demonstrating one-year remission or improvement of diabetes in 40% to 75% of patients who underwent a SG or an AGB [12, 13]. SG is an alternative procedure to RYGB for patients with BMI <50, the extremes of ages, and smokers.

In addition to glycemic control, improvement in distal peripheral neuropathy was identified following RYGB. An improvement or normalization of the Neuropathy Symptom Score (NSS) and the Neuropathy Deficit Score (NDS) in all patients has been found [14].

Hypertension

The association between obesity and the development of hypertension is well established. Weight loss, whether by an intensive lifestyle-medical modification program or by a bariatric operation, improves obesity-linked hypertension or contributes to remission. Patients undergoing a bariatric surgery plus intensive lifestyle medical management were able to achieve a similar reduction in systolic blood pressure at 12 months compared with patients managed with lifestyle medical modification alone [15]. While intensive lifestyle modification resulting in weight loss appears beneficial for resolution of hypertension, this is unfortunately not feasible for all patients, due to reasons such as lack of motivation or inability to exercise.

Data are unclear as to whether or not RYGB offers the highest resolution or reduction of hypertension of bariatric operations, as illustrated by several studies [16].

Dyslipidemia

Obesity-linked dyslipidemia is a well-established risk factor for cardiovascular disease [17]. The most commonly encountered dyslipidemias in obese individuals include hypertriglyceridemia, decreased HDL-cholesterol values, and increased LDL-cholesterol particles [18]. Multiple studies have demonstrated improved lipid profiles following bariatric procedures. The most extensively studied procedure is the RYGB. Mean total cholesterol levels decreased by 16%, triglyceride levels decreased by 63%, LDL- cholesterol levels decreased by 31%, total cholesterol/HDL-cholesterol risk ratio decreased by 60%, and HDL-cholesterol levels increased by 39%. In addition, over 80% of patients requiring lipid lowering medications preoperatively, no longer required medical therapy [19]. Malabsorptive procedures obtain at least similar results of improvement of dyslipidemia. A recent study of our group has demonstrated that after SG, HDL-cholesterol values increase and Triglycerides levels decreased significantly. However, total and LDL-cholesterol remained unaltered of present nonsignificant improvements. Notwithstanding, mainly based on the HDL-cholesterol increase, the cardiovascular risk index present a significant improvement after surgery [2].

Predictive Markers of Obesity and Cardiovascular Disease in Morbidly Obese Patients

BMI and Adiposity

In the 19th century, Adolphe Quetelet observed that the relative weight of the human was proportional to the square of the height. This relation was denominated Quetelet Index and later on, Body Mass Index (BMI) [20, 21]. The cut-off points of the BMI are very useful for epidemiological studies, but it does not represent an accurate measure of the body composition. Frequently, it underestimates obese subjects as just overweight ones. Based on a study performed on more than 6.000 subjects, investigators of the University Clinic of Navarra (Spain) developed an equation to calculate the body fat percentage, also known as adiposity, without depending on sophisticated technology and just based on anthropometric values easily obtained [22, 23]. The new formula, also known as CUN-BAE (Clínica Universidad de Navarra-Body Adiposity Estimator) is an approach to the fat composition and classifies it according previously established ranges. With this new classification, it has been demonstrated that subjects considered as lean or with overweight (BMI<30 Kg/m^2) in reality present elevated adiposity ranges, which might explain certain comorbidities associated with the metabolic syndrome [22].

Several studies have analyzed the impact of adiposity on cardiovascular risk, realizing that BMI associated or not to the waist circumference is less effective than adiposity determination [23, 24]. However, the actual devices to measure adiposity (bioelectric impedance, hydrostatic weight, pletismography, double-energy X-ray absorciometry, …) are often not available in all media, the measures are estimative and imply elevated sanitary costs [25, 26].

CUN-BAE formula has exposed that nearly one third of subjects classified as lean by the BMI, present an elevated adiposity, and 80% of patients classified as overweight, are really obese ones [22-24].

Thus, BMI does not define the obesity grade as an excess of adiposity, but a weight excess, without discriminating between fat, water and muscle. Despite BMI and adiposity present a certain degree of correlation, it is only moderate in morbidly obese patients before undergoing bariatric surgery and slightly increases in postoperative determinations. The effectiveness of bariatric surgery is not just limited to the reduction of body adiposity, but, when achieving it, the risk of suffering a cardiovascular event is also reduced [27].

Framingham Score and Castelli Index

In our medium, there are two indices, predictive of cardiovascular risk: Triglycerides/HDL-cholesterol (TG/HDL) ratio (Castelli Index) and the Framingham score, which analyzes age, gender, total cholesterol, HDL-cholesterol, tobacco habit and systolic arterial pressure. It has been considered that Framingham score is the most accurate method to calculate the cardiovascular risk, but its application is more complex than other scores [27]. Therefore, the TG/HDL index is preferred by many clinicians, as it can be numerically quantified and is not expressed as the probability of suffering a cardiovascular event, like the Framingham score. Diverse studies have shown that a TG/HDL index >3 is associated with increased cardiovascular risk. A previous study of our group has demonstrated that TG/HDL index correlates with the adiposity grade before and after bariatric surgery, but it does not correlate with BMI at any state. This reflects that both, adiposity and TG/HDL index, are better predictors of cardiovascular risk than BMI [4, 28, 29].

Serum Cortisol

Cortisol plays a role in the adiposity and finally in obesity development. Circulating serum levels of cortisol are higher among obese subjects with or without metabolic syndrome, than in lean ones. Cortisol induces the differentiation and proliferation of human adipocytes and their receptors are more profuse in the visceral adipose tissue than in the subcutaneous one. Moreover, cortisol contributes to the distribution of the fat from the peripherical depots to the central ones; it activates lipolysis and the release of free fatty acids to the blood circulation, increasing the risk of ateromatosis and consequently, the cardiovascular risk.

Weight loss reduces the serum cortisol levels down to normal ranges. According to this, cortisol levels might be considered as reflection of cardiovascular disease. Previous studies of our group demonstrated that the decrease in the adiposity directly correlates with the reduction in the cortisol levels. From the 6th month, the decrease in serum cortisol correlates with a reduction in the cardiovascular risk [2, 4, 30, 31]. All these data confirm the hypothesis that cortisol is an accurate predictor of cardiovascular risk in morbidly obese patients undergoing bariatric surgery.

Vitamin D

In the last decade, actions of vitamin D different than those related with the bone metabolism, have been discovered. These actions have been denominated as non-calcemic actions. These findings demonstrate that vitamin D has diverse functions, corresponding to a hormone rather than an inert vitamin [32, 33].

Deficiencies in vitamin D in obese patients are associated with metabolic syndrome and disorders in lipid levels (cholesterol and triglycerides). This suggests that vitamin D is a modifiable factor amenable for correction, which may imply a benefit in the cardiovascular risk of these patients [30].

Vitamin D stores mostly in the adipose tissue in obese patients, leading often to a secondary hyperparathyroidism. As they lose weight, the serum values of vitamin D increase. This explains the inverse correlation between the adiposity reduction and the increase of plasmatic levels of vitamin D after bariatric surgery [30].

REFERENCES

[1] Encinosa, WE; Bernard, DM; Du, D; Steiner, CA. Recent improvements in bariatric surgery outcomes. *Med Care*, 2009, 47, 531-5.

[2] Ruiz-Tovar, J; Oller, I; Tomas, A; et al. Midterm impact of sleeve gastrectomy, calibrated with a 50-Fr bougie, on weight loss, glucose hemostasis, lipid profiles and comorbidities in morbidly obese patients. *Am Surg*, 2012, 78, 969-74.

[3] Schauer, PR; Kashyap, SR; Wolski, K; et al. Bariatric surgery versus intensive medical therapy in obese patients with diabetes. *N Engl J Med*, 2012, 366, 1567-76.

[4] Zubiaga, L; Ruiz-Tovar, J; Diez-Tabernilla, M; et al. Fórmula CUN-BAE y factores bioquímicos como marcadores predictivos de obesidad y enfermedad cardiovascular en pacientes pre y post gastrectomía vertical. *Nutr Hosp*, 2014, 30, 281-6.

[5] Rubino, F. Is type 2 diabetes an operable intestinal disease? A provocative yet reasonable hypothesis. *Diabetes Care*, 2008, 31, Suppl 2, S290-6.

[6] Schauer, PR; Kashyap, SR; Wolski, K; et al. Bariatric surgery versus intensive medical therapy in obese patients with diabetes. *N Engl J Med*, 2012, 366, 1567-76.

[7] Mingrone, G; Panunzi, S; De Gaetano, A; et al. Bariatric surgery versus conventional medical therapy for type 2 diabetes. *N Engl J Med*, 2012, 366, 1577-85.

[8] Ikramuddin, S; Korner, J; Lee, WJ; et al. Roux-en-Y gastric bypass vs intensive medical management for the control of type 2 diabetes, hypertension, and hyperlipidemia: the Diabetes Surgery Study randomized clinical trial. *JAMA*, 2013, 309, 2240-9.

[9] Rubino, F; Kaplan, LM; Schauer, PR; et al. The Diabetes Surgery Summit consensus conference: recommendations for the evaluation and use of gastrointestinal surgery to treat type 2 diabetes mellitus. *Ann Surg*, 2010, 251, 399-405.

[10] Kenngott, HG; Clemens, G; Gondan, M; et al. DiaSurg 2 trial - surgical vs. medical treatment of insulin-dependent type 2 diabetes mellitus in patients with a body mass index between 26 and 35 kg/m2: study protocol of a randomized controlled multicenter trial - DRKS00004550. *Trials*, 2013, 14, 183.

[11] Hutter, MM; Schirmer, BD; Jones, DB; et al. First report from the American College of Surgeons Bariatric Surgery Center Network: laparoscopic sleeve gastrectomy has morbidity and effectiveness positioned between the band and the bypass. *Ann Surg*, 2011, 254, 410-20.

[12] Dixon, JB; O'Brien, PE; Playfair, J; et al. Adjustable gastric banding and conventional therapy for type 2 diabetes: a randomized controlled trial. *JAMA*, 2008, 299, 316-23.

[13] Ahn, SM; Pomp, A; Rubino, F. Metabolic surgery for type 2 diabetes. *Ann N Y Acad Sci*, 2010, 1212, E37-45.

[14] Müller-Stich, BP; Fischer, L; Kenngott, HG; et al. Gastric bypass leads to improvement of diabetic neuropathy independent of glucose normalization--results of a prospective cohort study (DiaSurg 1 study). *Ann Surg*, 2013, 258, 760-5.

[15] Ikramuddin, S; Korner, J; Lee, WJ; et al. Roux-en-Y gastric bypass vs intensive medical management for the control of type 2 diabetes, hypertension, and hyperlipidemia: the Diabetes Surgery Study randomized clinical trial. *JAMA*, 2013, 309, 2240-9.

[16] Zhang, N; Maffei, A; Cerabona, T; et al. Reduction in obesity-related comorbidities: is gastric bypass better than sleeve gastrectomy? *Surg Endosc*, 2013, 27, 1273-80.

[17] Anderson, KM; Castelli, WP; Levy, D. Cholesterol and mortality. 30 years of follow-up from the Framingham study. *JAMA*, 1987, 257, 2176-80.

[18] Joshi, AV; Day, D; Lubowski, TJ; Ambegaonkar, A. Relationship between obesity and cardiovascular risk factors: findings from a multi-state screening project in the United States. *Curr Med Res Opin*, 2005, 21, 1755-61.

[19] Nguyen, NT; Varela, E; Sabio, A; et al. Resolution of hyperlipidemia after laparoscopic Roux-en-Y gastric bypass. *J Am Coll Surg*, 2006, 203, 24-9.

[20] Frühbeck, G; Diez-Caballero, A; Gómez-Ambrosi, J; et al. Preventing obesity. Doctors underestimate obesity. *BMJ*, 2003, 326, 102-3.

[21] Frühbeck, G. Screening and interventions for obesity in adults. *Ann Intern Med*, 2004, 141, 245-6.

[22] Gómez-Ambrosi, J; Silva, C; Catalán, V; et al. Clinical usefulness of a new equation for estimating body fat. *Diabetes Care*, 2012,2,383-8.

[23] Catalán, V; Gómez-Ambrosi, J; Ramírez, B; et al. Proinflammatory cytokines in obesity: impact of type 2 diabetes mellitus and gastric bypass. *Obes Surg*, 2007, 17, 1464-74.

[24] Catalán, V; Gómez-Ambrosi, J; Rodríguez, A; et al. Increased circulating and visceral adipose tissue expression levels of YKL-40 in obesity-associated type 2 diabetes are related to inflammation: impact of conventional weight loss and gastric bypass. *J Clin Endocrinol Metab*, 2011, 96, 200-9.

[25] Flegal, KM; Shepherd, JA; Looker, AC; et al. Comparisons of percentage body fat, body mass index, waist circumference, and waist-stature ratio in adults. *Am J Clin Nutr*, 2009, 89, 500-8.

[26] Basterra, FJ; Bes, M; Segui, M; Forga, L; Martínez, JA; Martínez, MA. Tendencias de la obesidad, diabetes mellitus, hipertensión e hipercolesterolemia en España, 1997-2003. *Med Clin (Barc)*, 2007, 129, 405-8.

[27] Fields, DA; Goran, MI; McCrory, MA. Body-composition assessment via air-displacement plethysmography in adults and children: A review. *Am J Clin Nutr*, 2002, 75, 453-67.

[28] Carbajo, MA; Castro, MJ; Kleinfinger, S; et al. Effects of a balanced energy and high protein formula diet (Vegestart complet®) *vs.* low-calorie regular diet in morbid obese patients prior to bariatric surgery (laparoscopic single anastomosis gastric bypass): A prospective, double-blind randomized study. *Nutr Hosp*, 2010, 25 (6), 939-48.

[29] O'Donnela, C; Elosuab, R. Factores de riesgo cardiovascular. Perspectivas derivadas del Framingham Heart Study. *Rev Esp Cardiol*, 2008, 61, 299-310.

[30] Ruiz-Tovar, J; Oller, I; Galindo, I; et al. Change in Levels of C-Reactive Protein (CRP) and Serum Cortisol in Morbidly Obese Patients After Laparoscopic Sleeve Gastrectomy. *Obes Surg*, 2013, 23, 764-9.

[31] Frankenfield, DC; Rowe, WA; Cooney, RN; et al. Limits of body mass index to detect obesity and predict body composition. *Nutrition*, 2001, 17, 26-30.

[32] Clare-Grace, PD; Vincent, R; Aylwin, SJ. High prevalence of vitamin D insufficiency in a United Kingdom urban morbidly obese population: implications for testing and treatment. *Surg Obes Relat Dis*, 2013, 29. pii:S1550-7289(13)00257-8.

[33] Ruiz-Tovar, J; Oller, I; Tomas, A; et al. Mid-term effects of sleeve gastrectomy on calcium metabolism parameters. Vitamin D and parathormone (PTH) in morbid obese women. *Obes Surg*, 2012, 22 (5), 797-801.

In: A Closer Look at Cardiovascular … ISBN: 978-1-53613-939-6
Editor: Faris van Kilsdonk

Chapter 5

Gender Differences in Cardiovascular Diseases and Their Risk Factors

Toralben Patel, MD, MPH
Cardiac and Vascular Consultants,
Lecanto, FL, US

Abstract

Cardiovascular diseases (CVD) are the leading cause of death in both men and women. There has been steady decline in mortality from CVD in middle-aged men (35 to 54 years) based on recent data from the National Health and Nutrition Examination Surveys (NHANES) but for women this rate has remained relatively unchanged. Although there are similarities in most classic risk factors in men and women, there are varying implications of these risk factors for both genders. Because of higher proportion of women in aging population with higher expression of cardiovascular risk factors, each year more women than men die because of CVD. There is increased prevalence of risk factors for heart disease in women such as obesity, smoking and diabetes and it is likely responsible for increasing burden of heart disease in women of young age. This increased risk is often under recognized because of misperception of protective effect of female hormones. Clear sex differences have been described in the epidemiology, pathophysiology, clinical presentation of disease, prevalence of risk factors and response to diagnostic tests. Furthermore, several risk factors that solely affect women include oral contraceptives, hormone replacement therapy, pregnancy-related heart disease and menopausal status. Females are also significantly under represented in cardiovascular clinical trials. Newer studies have noted marked sex difference in cardiovascular outcomes in preventive strategies and effects of therapy.

In spite of the growing evidence of magnitude of heart disease in women, they are still evaluated less intensively; risk is often undermined, under referred for diagnostic testing and not treated as aggressively as men. Increasing awareness and identification of gender based differences in cardiovascular risk factors needs more attention, which should result in a better primary and secondary prevention of cardiovascular events.

1. Introduction

Cardiovascular diseases spectrum includes the following four prime areas:

- Coronary Heart disease manifested as angina pectoris, congestive heart failure, myocardial infarction (MI) and cardiac death.
- Cerebrovascular disease manifested as transient ischemic attack and stroke.
- Peripheral vascular disease manifested by intermittent claudication, resting pain, gangrene and occasionally loss of limb.
- Aortic disorders manifested by aortic atherosclerosis, thoracic and abdominal aortic aneurysm.

Cardiovascular diseases although previously considered predominantly "male" disease, is now known to be responsible for death of one in three females [1]. It is the leading cause of death in women in both industrialized and developing world exceeding deaths from all cancers combined [2]. Notwithstanding improvement in cardiovascular outcomes in the last decade, substantial gender disparities are evident. Recent data suggest in fact increasing burden of cardiovascular diseases in young women [1, 3]. The disturbingly increased incidence of diabetes, obesity, physical inactivity and other comorbid conditions entrenches surge of cardiovascular diseases.

Many biologic and environmental factors, including sex hormones, plays a role in difference in cardiovascular diseases between men and women [4]. Although overall incidence of myocardial infarction is lower in women as compared to men, incidence of myocardial infarction dramatically increases in postmenopausal women [5]. But the clear role of menopause and sex hormones is not evident. Premenopausal females presenting with myocardial infarction have worse prognosis [6, 7]. Females present with more atypical symptoms, have more unrecognized MIs and less likely to receive invasive and standard of care treatment [8, 9]. Anatomically, females have higher occurrence of non-obstructive coronary heart disease, microvascular disease, endothelial dysfunction and stress induced cardiomyopathy. Discrepancies are also noted in risk factor profile between males and females. Females although more likely to maintain ideal body weight, are not as much physically active as males [10].

Cardiovascular diseases are majorly preventable and risk factor reduction has contributed to overall decline in rates of coronary heart diseases [1, 11]. However, this decline is slower for women as compared to men and so it is imperative to have thorough understanding of these risk factors to modify this gender based outcomes gap [1, 3]. An overview of the determinants of cardiovascular risk in women will be reviewed here highlighting gender specific factors.

2. Cardiovascular Risk Factors Common in Men and Women

2.1. Non Modifiable Cardiovascular Risk Factors

2.1.1. Age

Age is the major non-modifiable cardiovascular risk factor for cardiovascular disorders in both genders. Age by itself also contributes to development of CVD. Savji et al. studied the relationship between vascular disease in different arterial territories and advanced age in a population database of over 3.6 million subjects [12]. Between 2003 and 2008, over 3.6 million subjects self-referred for screening ankle brachial indices <0.9 for peripheral artery disease (PAD), and ultrasound imaging for carotid artery stenosis (CAS) > 50% and abdominal aortic aneurysm (AAA) > 3 cm. Prevalence of any vascular disease increased with advanced age after adjusting for traditional risk factors (40 to 50 years: 2%, 51 to 60 years: 3.5%, 61 to 70 years: 7.1%, 71 to 80 years: 13.0%, 81 to 90 years: 22.3%, 91 to 100 years: 32.5%; $p < 0.0001$). Each additional decade of life was associated with an approximate doubling of the risk of vascular disease (the odds of PAD (odds ratio [OR]: 2.14; 95% confidence interval [CI]: 2.12 to 2.15), CAS (OR: 1.80; 95% CI: 1.79 to 1.81), and AAA (OR: 2.33; 95% CI: 2.30 to 2.36).

2.1.2. Family History

Family history of premature coronary heart disease is an independent risk factor for CHD especially in young individuals [13, 14]. Family history is defined variably in different studies. In general most commonly used definition is development of coronary heart disease, MI or sudden death in father or first degree male relative at age less than 55 years, or mother or first degree female relative at age less than 65 years [15].

Family history is recommended for risk stratification in major cardiovascular risk prediction models. Family history of premature cardiovascular disease increased risk of developing coronary heart disease by mostly 40-60 percent in large cohort studies [10]. Family history increased risk of cardiac event more in women as compared to men [16, 17].

2.2. Modifiable Cardiovascular Risk Factors

2.2.1. Hyperlipidemia

Hyperlipidemia has been shown to increase risk of cardiovascular disease and cardiovascular events based on numerous epidemiologic studies and randomized controlled trials [18]. There is a difference in role of different lipoprotein factors in risk stratification in women as compared to men. Biologically, estrogen decreases total cholesterol and low-density lipoprotein (LDL) by increasing hepatic expression of lipoproteins and increases high-density lipoprotein (HDL) and triglycerides [19]. During early postmenopausal period and peri-menopausal period there is modest increase in serum lipids especially LDL and triglycerides [20]. Hypertriglyceridemia results in significantly increased coronary risk in women as compared to men [21, 22]. Furthermore, low HDL, non-HDL cholesterol (total cholesterol minus HDL cholesterol level) and ratio of total cholesterol to HDL cholesterol level are better predictors of future cardiovascular events as compared to other lipoprotein factors [23, 24]. Mainstay of therapy for hyperlipidemia is lifestyle modification and pharmacologic therapy with statins for primary prevention. The data for primary prevention with statin therapy is based on multiple randomized control trials, although efficacy of statin in women has been questioned because of underrepresentation of females in these trials. In contrast, women benefit from statin therapy for secondary prevention more than men in terms of regression of coronary lesions (25-27). Furthermore, in recent meta-analysis, efficacy of statin for primary prevention has found to be equal in men and women [28, 29].

2.2.2. Hypertension

Hypertension is one of the strongest predictor for almost all different cardiovascular diseases acquired during life across all ages [16, 23]. Postmenopausal women have significantly increased prevalence of high blood pressure [30].

In older women, hypertension as compared to men is a strong predictor of cardiovascular risk and also is noted to be associated with coronary heart disease. However, high blood pressure is associated with 10-fold increase in mortality in younger premenopausal patients [31]. In addition, there are also significant ethnic disparities noted in blood pressure. White male and females have lower blood pressure as compared to black males and females [30]. In fact, approximately 75% of African American women over age 75 suffer from hypertension [32].

Adequate control of blood pressure is known to improve survival. There is no significant gender difference in effect of antihypertensive therapies, antihypertensive agents and recommended target for blood pressure values. However, when recommending specific antihypertensive agent other comorbidities and reproductive health should be taken into consideration.

2.2.3. Diabetes

When it comes to cardiovascular diseases, there is very little uncertainty that diabetes is of utmost significance. Diabetes is considered significant predictor of cardiovascular risk and prognosis in both men and women [16, 23]. The number of people affected with diabetes has almost quadrupled from 5.5 million in 1980 to 23.1 million in 2015 [10, 33]. By 2050, it is estimated that the prevalence of diabetes will be doubled and the number of women affected with diabetes will be higher than men [10, 34]. The National Cholesterol Education Program (NCEP) Adult treatment panel (ATP) III Guidelines in 2001 recommended that diabetes be considered as "coronary heart disease risk equivalent" [15]. The increased CHD risk is higher in women with diabetes as compared to men [35-37]. Huskey et al. in a meta-analysis of 37 studies involving 450,000 patients showed that women have double the risk of fatal coronary heart disease as compared to men along with poor quality of life [35]. The relative higher risk in females is due to presence of other comorbidities and also lack of optimal treatment of diabetes and other modifiable risk factors [36, 37]. Additionally, insulin resistant states such as polycystic ovarian disease carries increased cardiovascular risk for females [35].

2.2.4. Lifestyle Related Risk Factors

2.2.4.1. Smoking

Smoking causes more deaths from coronary heart disease and stroke than any other cause [2, 38]. Cigarette smoking is on the major lifestyle risk factor for development of atherosclerosis [40]. Smoking not only increases development of atherosclerosis, coronary heart disease but also increases risk of acute thrombosis [39]. The mechanism of smoking related cardiovascular risk is thought to be due to increased inflammation and oxidation of LDL [40]. Females who smoke are at 25% higher risk of developing coronary heart disease as compared to males [41]. According to current data, smoking is becoming more prevalent in younger women and it is most important risk factor for sudden cardiac death [39]. Additionally, a large prospective study has confirmed relationship between smoking and diabetes. Females who smoked > 2 packs/day had 74% higher rate of diabetes than female who did not smoke. The corresponding increase for men was only 45% [42].

Smoking cessation has favorable decrease in morbidity and mortality from cardiovascular events. Cessation of smoking in women is associated with rapid decline in cardiovascular risk. Rosenberg et al. found that females who have quit smoking for 3 or more years have similar risk of myocardial infarction compared with females who never smoked [43]. However, females are less successful than males in quitting smoking. Also women and young smoker do not receive adequate counseling on smoking cessation as compared to men and older smokers [10, 44].

Epidemiologic studies have shown that passive smoking is also associated with increased cardiovascular risk. Wells et al. showed that females exposed to passive smoking at workplace have increased morbidity and mortality from cardiovascular disease [45].

2.2.4.2. Obesity

Obesity is defined as body mass index (BMI) more than 30. The United States and other countries are experiencing an epidemic of obesity. From 1996 to 2000, rates of obesity in women have significantly increased from 16% to 34% as compared to men 11% to 28% [46, 47]. Obesity has been now recognized as a disease by American Medical Association, requiring treatment and prevention efforts [48]. There is a strong relationship between obesity and traditional cardiovascular risk factors [49-51]. There is higher prevalence of hypertension, diabetes and low HDL in obese patients [49-51]. A Large prospective Nurses Health Study of over 115000 women showed increasing cardiovascular mortality and all cause mortality with increasing BMI [52]. The American Heart Association recommends to keep BMI < 25 kg/m^2, although there is no significant studies showing that weight loss improves long term cardiovascular outcomes.

2.2.4.3. Physical Inactivity

Physical inactivity is an established risk factor for cardiovascular diseases [53]. There is a prominent dose response relationship between cardiovascular disease related mortality, morbidity and physical activity. Although, even mild to moderate physical activity has been shown to be protective [54, 55]. Women and men have similar cardiovascular risk reduction by engaging in regular physical activity. An observational Study of over 70,000 postmenopausal women showed that prolonged sitting predicted an increase in cardiovascular risk. Furthermore, study found that both walking and vigorous activities were associated with reduction in cardiovascular risk in postmenopausal women irrespective of race, ethnic group, age or body mass index [56]. However, there is significant decline in physical activities in women and corresponding increase in obesity [57].

2.2.4.4. Alcohol Intake

Over the past several decades, many published studies have shown that mild to moderate alcohol intake has been associated with lower mortality due to heart disease [58]. However, heavier amount of alcohol intake can increase triglycerides; promote physical inactivity, cause weight gain and increased incidence of hypertension [59]. In addition, Fuchs et al. demonstrated that higher intake of alcohol in women also increases death from breast cancer and cirrhosis and counters the cardio protective effect [60].

2.2.4.5. Psycho-Social Factors

Psychosocial factors such, as stress has been associated with increased cardiovascular risk and poor prognosis in women [61, 62]. Young women are at higher risk of depression after an acute myocardial infarction [63]. The American Heart Association recommends that depression be recognized as a risk factor for increased cardiovascular risk like hypertension, diabetes. A study done in postmenopausal women found depression to be an independent predictor of death [62]. Depression has been shown to increase risk of behavioral changes leading to unhealthy lifestyle such as consuming a diet rich in saturated fat and calories, smoking, decreased physical activity and decreased medication follow up compliance [64-67]. Furthermore, the biological and chemical factors that trigger mental health issues also could influence heart disease.

2.2.5. Inflammatory Markers

There is a significant role of inflammation in pathogenesis of atherosclerosis [68]. Inflammatory disorders such as rheumatoid arthritis, lupus and chronic obstructive lung disease have increased cardiovascular events [69, 70]. Different inflammatory risk markers have been studied for increased cardiovascular risk [71]. Most widely studied C- reactive protein was found to be strong and independent predictor of cardiovascular disease based on Women's Health Study [72]. However, there is very minimal use of inflammatory markers in routine clinical practice.

2.2.6. Chronic Kidney Disease

Chronic kidney disease (CKD) is a predictor of increased cardiovascular events and mortality in both genders independent of traditional cardiovascular risk factors [73]. Even mild kidney disease is associated with increased cardiovascular risk. Women with diabetes are at 35% increased risk of developing CKD compared with men, which can likely predisposing them to higher cardiovascular risk [74].

2.2.7. Others

There is increased in cardiovascular risk with elevated fibrinogen levels in both men and women [75]. Also albuminuria, a marker of arterial wall damage, is associated with increased cardiovascular events [76].

Hyperhomocysteinemia have also been associated with increased cardiovascular risk in both genders [77].

3. Cardiovascular Risk Factors Specific to Women

3.1. Menopause and Hormone Replacement Therapy

There is a significant increase in incidence of cardiovascular disease in postmenopausal women [1]. Conventionally premenopausal women are considered at lower risk of cardiovascular disease because of cardioprotective effect of female hormones [5]. Females are a decade older when diagnosed with CHD and it is associated with beneficial effect of premenopausal state. Menopause is associated with lot of biologic changes including gradual decline in estrogen. Menopause, if itself is a risk factor or a marker increased risk is still controversial and there is conflicting data in current existing literature.

The American College of Cardiology/American Heart Association (ACC/AHA) guidelines identify menopause as a risk factor for cardiovascular diseases [1]. Early menopause either natural or surgical has been positively associated with increased cardiovascular risk [78-80]. However, causal role of menopause in increasing cardiovascular risk is not explicit. Howard et al. showed that hysterectomy with or without oophorectomy is not associated with increased cardiovascular risk [81]. There is increasing school of thought that there is a continuum of risk and menopause is just a risk marker, rather than a risk factor. Furthermore, supporting this theory is notable lack of cardiovascular risk reduction with hormone replacement therapy in post-menopausal women in randomized control trials. Women's Health Initiative study showed increased harm with hormone replacement therapy [82-84]. Postmenopausal women have increased incidence of traditional cardiac risk factors, which puts them at increased cardiovascular risk [81]. In conjunction of these findings, the

American College of Cardiology/American Heart Association guidelines and United States Preventive Service Task Force recommend against hormone replacement therapy for primary and secondary cardiovascular disease prevention.

3.2. Menarche

Early menarche is associated with increased cardiovascular risk [85-87]. Canoy et al. showed that women who have menarche at age 10 have increased cardiovascular risk as compared to women who experienced menarche at age 13 [85]. A systematic review and meta-analysis of six smaller studies supported this finding by demonstrating that for each year increase in age of menarche was associated with reduction in mortality [86].

3.3. Oral Contraceptives

Oral contraceptives are associated with increased cardiovascular risk [88-90]. This is seen especially in young female who are smokers [89, 90].

3.4. Pregnancy Related Disorders

Women who develop preeclampsia and gestational diabetes are not only at increased risk of developing hypertension and diabetes respectively later in life but also with associated increased cardiovascular risk [91, 92].

Women with recurrent spontaneous pregnancy loss are at increased risk of myocardial infarction later in life [93]. This risk may be attributed to increase in inflammatory mediators associated with underlying condition and probably also associated procoagulant state. Additionally, women who deliver preterm babies are at increased cardiovascular risk [94].

4. Cardiovascular Risk Stratification in Women

Several different risk scores have been developed to predict cardiovascular outcomes. The Framingham risk score is the most commonly used score to estimate risk of cardiovascular events over 10 years [95, 96]. The Framingham risk score is known to underestimate risk in women [97]. Whereas, Reynolds risk score was developed specifically to estimate cardiovascular risk in women. It incorporates conventional cardiovascular risk factors in addition to family history and C-reactive protein. It is better validated than Framingham risk score and also improved overall discrimination overall and in black and white women [97]. The 2013 American College of Cardiology/American Heart Association risk calculator also incorporated stroke as combined endpoint in atherosclerotic cardiovascular disease (ASCVD), which is particularly important in women, because rates of stroke in women can be as high as those for myocardial infarction [98].

There are advantages and disadvantages associated with any risk prediction models. No model is appropriate for all and also the cardiovascular risk is dynamic rather than static. The approach for cardiovascular risk prediction should be individualized based on patient specific characteristics [99].

Conclusion

While there has been major decline in overall cardiovascular mortality, this rate of decline has been slower for women as compared to men and especially in young women. Increasing awareness and identification of gender-based differences in cardiovascular risk factors needs more attention to bridge the gender gap in cardiovascular outcomes.

REFERENCES

[1] Mosca L., Benjamin E.J., Berra K. et al., Effectiveness-based guidelines for the prevention of cardiovascular disease in women–2011 update: a guideline from the American Heart Association. *Circulation.* 123 (11), 1243–1262 (2011).

[2] GBD 2013 Mortality and Causes of Death Collaborators. Global, regional, and national age-sex specific all-cause and cause-specific mortality for 240 causes of death, 1990-2013: a systematic analysis for the Global Burden of Disease Study. *Lancet.* 385 (9963), 117 - 171 (2015).

[3] Ford E.S., Capewell S., Coronary heart disease mortality among young adults in the US from 1980 through 2002: concealed leveling of mortality rates. *J. Am. Coll. Cardiol.* 50(22), 2128–2132 (2007).

[4] Luczak E.D., Leinwand L.A., Sex-based cardiac physiology. *Ann. Rev. Physiol.* 71, 1–18 (2009).

[5] Lerner D.J., Kannel W.B., Patterns of coronary heart disease morbidity and mortality in the sexes: a 26-year follow-up of the Framingham population. *Am Heart J.* 111 (2), 383 – 390 (1986).

[6] Ford E.S., Ajani U.A., Croft J.B. et al., Explaining the decrease in US deaths from coronary disease, 1980–2000. N. *Engl. J. Med.* 356(23), 2388–2398 (2007).

[7] Wenger N.K., You've come a long way, baby: cardiovascular health and disease in women: problems and prospects. *Circulation.* 109(5), 558–560 (2004).

[8] Shlipak M.G., Elmouchi D.A., Herrington D.M. et al., The incidence of unrecognized myocardial infarction in women with coronary heart disease. *Ann. Intern. Med.* 134(11), 1043–1047 (2001).

[9] Rathore S.S., Chen J., Wang Y., Radford M.J., Vaccarino V., Krumholz H.M., Sex differences in cardiac catheterization: the role of physician gender. *JAMA.* 286(22), 2849–2856 (2001).

[10] Go A.S., Mozaffarian D., Roger V.L. et al., Heart disease and stroke statistics – 2013 update: a report from the American Heart Association. *Circulation.* 127(1), e6–e245 (2013).

[11] Hu F.B., Stampfer M.J., Manson J.E., et al., Trends in the incidence of coronary heart disease and changes in diet and lifestyle in women. *N Engl J Med*. 343 (8), 530- 537(2000).

[12] Savji N., Rockman C.B., Skolnick A.H. et al. Association between advanced age and vascular disease in different arterial territories: a population database of over 3.6 million subjects. *J Am Coll Cardiol*. 61(16), 1736 - 1743 (2013).

[13] Marenberg M.E., Risch N., Berkman L.F., Floderus B., de Faire U., Genetic susceptibility to death from coronary heart disease in a study of twins. *N. Engl. J. Med.* 330(15), 1041–1046 (1994).

[14] Parikh N.I., Hwang S.J., Larson M.G., et al. Parental occurrence of premature cardiovascular disease predicts increased coronary artery and abdominal aortic calcification in the Framingham Offspring and Third Generation cohorts. *Circulation*. 116 (13), 1473–1481 (2007).

[15] National Cholesterol Education Program (NCEP) Expert Panel on Detection, Evaluation, and Treatment of High Blood Cholesterol in Adults (Adult Treatment Panel III). Third Report of the National Cholesterol Education Program (NCEP) Expert Panel on Detection, Evaluation, and Treatment of High Blood Cholesterol in Adults (Adult Treatment Panel III) final report. *Circulation*. 106(25), 3143–3421 (2002).

[16] Sullivan A.K., Holdright D.R., Wright C.A., et al. Chest pain in women: clinical, investigative, and prognostic features. *BMJ*. 308 (6933), 883-886 (1994).

[17] Ridker P.M., Buring J.E., Rifai N., Cook N.R., Development and validation of improved algorithms for the assessment of global cardiovascular risk in women: the Reynolds Risk Score. *JAMA*. 297 (6), 611 – 619 (2007).

[18] Steinberg D., Thematic review series: the pathogenesis of atherosclerosis. An interpretive history of the cholesterol controversy: Part I. *J. Lipid Res*. 45(9), 1583–1593 (2004).

[19] Mendelsohn M.E., Karas R.H., The protective effects of estrogen on the cardiovascular system. *N. Engl. J. Med*. 340(23), 1801–1811 (1999).

[20] Derby C.A., Crawford S.L., Pasternak R.C., Sowers M., Sternfeld B., Matthews K.A., Lipid changes during the menopause transition in relation to age and weight: the Study of Women's Health Across the Nation. *Am. J. Epidemiol.* 169(11), 1352–1361 (2009).

[21] Stock E.O., Redberg R., Cardiovascular disease in women. *Curr. Prob. Cardiol.* 37(11), 450–526 (2012).

[22] Ridker P.M., Rifai N., Cook N.R., Bradwin G., Buring J.E., Non-HDL cholesterol, apolipoproteins A-I and B100, standard lipid measures, lipid ratios, and CRP as risk factors for cardiovascular disease in women. *JAMA*. 294(3), 326–333 (2005).

[23] Rich-Edwards J.W., Manson J.E., Hennekens C.H., Buring J.E., The primary prevention of coronary heart disease in women. *N Engl J Med.* 332 (26), 1758 – 1766 (1995).

[24] Cholesterol Treatment Trialists' (CTT) Collaboration, Fulcher J., O'Connell R., et al. Efficacy and safety of LDL-lowering therapy among men and women: meta-analysis of individual data from 174,000 participants in 27 randomised trials. *Lancet.* 385 (9976), 1397-1405 (2015).

[25] Scandinavian Simvastatin Survival Study Group. Randomised trial of cholesterol lowering in 4444 patients with coronary heart disease: the Scandinavian Simvastatin Survival Study (4S). *Lancet*. 344 (8934), 1383 – 1389 (1994).

[26] Miettinen T.A., Pyörälä K., Olsson A.G. et al., Cholesterol-lowering therapy in women and elderly patients with myocardial infarction or angina pectoris: findings from the Scandinavian Simvastatin Survival Study (4S). *Circulation.* 96 (12), 4211 – 4218 (1997).

[27] Lewis S.J., Sacks F.M., Mitchell J.S. et al., Effect of pravastatin on cardiovascular events in women after myocardial infarction: the cholesterol and recurrent events (CARE) trial. *J Am Coll Cardiol*. 32 (1), 140-146 (1998).

[28] Kostis W.J., Cheng J.Q., Dobrzynski J.M. et al., Meta-analysis of statin effects in women versus men. *J Am Coll Cardiol*. 59 (6), 572 – 582 (2012).

[29] Kane J.P., Malloy M.J., Ports T.A. et al., Regression of coronary atherosclerosis during treatment of familial hypercholesterolemia with combined drug regimens. *JAMA*. 264 (23), 3007 – 3012 (1990).

[30] Wolz M., Cutler J., Roccella E.J., Rohde F., Thom T., Burt V., Statement from the National High Blood Pressure Education Program: prevalence of hypertension. *Am. J. Hypertens.* 13(1 Pt 1), 103–104 (2000).

[31] Cornoni-Huntley J., LaCroix A.Z., Havlik R.J., Race and sex differentials in the impact of hypertension in the United States. The National Health and Nutrition Examination Survey I Epidemiologic Follow-up Study. *Arch Intern Med.* 149 (4), 780 – 788 (1989).

[32] Narayan K.M., Boyle J.P., Geiss L.S., Saaddine J.B., Thompson T.J., Impact of recent increase in incidence on future diabetes burden: US, 2005–2050. *Diabetes Care*. 29(9), 2114–2116 (2006).

[33] Huxley R., Barzi F., Woodward M., Excess risk of fatal coronary heart disease associated with diabetes in men and women: meta-analysis of 37 prospective cohort studies. *BMJ.* 332(7533), 73–78 (2006).

[34] Centers for Disease Control and Prevention. Number (in Millions) of Civilian, *Non-institutionalized Adults with Diagnosed Diabetes*, United States, 1980-2015 (CDC website). 2015. Available at: https://www.cdc.gov/diabetes/data/index.html. Accessed on 4/25/18.

[35] Talbott E.O., Zborowski J.V., Rager J.R., Kip K.E., Xu X., Orchard TJ., Polycystic ovarian syndrome (PCOS): A significant contributor to the overall burden of Type 2 diabetes in women. *J. Womens Health*. 16(2), 191–197 (2007).

[36] Wexler D.J., Grant R.W., Meigs J.B., Nathan D.M., Cagliero E., Sex disparities in treatment of cardiac risk factors in patients with Type 2 diabetes. *Diabetes Care*. 28(3), 514–520 (2005).

[37] Weiner D.E., Tighiouart H., Amin M.G., et al. Chronic kidney disease as a risk factor for cardiovascular disease and all-cause mortality: a pooled analysis of community-based studies. *J Am Soc Nephrol.* 15(5), 1307–1315 (2004).

[38] Danaei G., Ding E.L., Mozaffarian D., et al. The preventable causes of death in the United States: comparative risk assessment of dietary, lifestyle, and metabolic risk factors. *PLoS Med.* 6(4), e1000058 (2009).

[39] Wells A.J., Heart disease from passive smoking in the workplace, *J Am Coll Cardiol.* 31 (1), 1-9 (1998).

[40] Ambrose J.A., Barua R.S., The pathophysiology of cigarette smoking and cardiovascular disease: an update. *J. Am. Coll. Cardiol.* 43(10), 1731–1737 (2004).

[41] Will J.C., Galuska D.A., Ford E.S., Mokdad A., Calle E.E., Cigarette smoking and diabetes mellitus: evidence of a positive association from a large prospective cohort study. *Int J Epidemiol.* 30 (3), 540-546 (2001).

[42] Rosenberg L., Palmer J.R., Shapiro S., Decline in the risk of myocardial infarction among women who stop smoking. *N Engl J Med.* 322(4), 213 – 217 (1990).

[43] Steliga M.A., Dresler C.M., Smoking cessation: crucial to target women as well as men. *Lancet.* 378(9799), 1278–1279 (2011).

[44] Mokdad A.H., Ford E.S., Bowman B.A., et al. Prevalence of obesity, diabetes, and obesity-related health risk factors. *JAMA*. 289(1), 76–79 (2003).

[45] Huxley R.R., Woodward M., Cigarette smoking as a risk factor for coronary heart disease in women compared with men: a systematic review and meta-analysis of prospective cohort studies. *Lancet.* 378(9799), 1297–1305 (2011).

[46] Truong K.D., Sturm R., Weight gain trends across sociodemographic groups in the United States. *Am J Public Health.* 95(9), 1602–1606 (2005).

[47] Li T.Y., Rana J.S., Manson J.E. et al., Obesity as compared with physical activity in predicting risk of coronary heart disease in women. *Circulation.* 113(4), 499–506 (2006).

[48] Pollack A., *A.M.A. Recognizes obesity as a disease.* [Internet]. 2013. Available from: http://www.nytimes.com/2013/06/19/business/ama-recognizes-obesity-as-a-disease.html.

[49] Freedman D.S., Khan L.K., Serdula M.K., Galuska D.A., Dietz W.H., Trends and correlates of class 3 obesity in the United States from 1990 through 2000. *JAMA.* 288(14), 1758–1761 (2002).

[50] Skyler J.S., Oddo C., Diabetes trends in the USA. *Diabetes Metab Res Rev.* 18(suppl 3), S21–S26 (2002).

[51] Gregg E.W., Cheng Y.J., Cadwell B.L., et al. Secular trends in cardiovascular disease risk factors according to body mass index in US adults. *JAMA.* 293(15), 1868–1874 (2005).

[52] King D.E., Mainous A.G. 3rd, Carnemolla M., Everett C.J., Adherence to healthy lifestyle habits in US adults, 1988–2006. *Am. J. Med.* 122(6), 528–534 (2009).

[53] Powell K.E., Thompson P.D., Caspersen C.J., Kendrick J.S., Physical activity and the incidence of coronary heart disease. *Annu Rev Public* Health. 8, 253-287 (1987).

[54] Tanasescu M., Leitzmann M.F., Rimm E.B. et al., Exercise type and intensity in relation to coronary heart disease in men. *JAMA.* 288 (16), 1994-2000 (2002).

[55] Lee D.C., Pate R.R., Lavie C.J. et al., Leisure-time running reduces all-cause and cardiovascular mortality risk. *J Am Coll Cardiol.* 64 (5), 472-481 (2014).

[56] Manson J.E., Greenland P., LaCroix A.Z. et al., Walking compared with vigorous exercise for the prevention of cardiovascular events in women. *N Engl J Med.* 347(10), 716-25 (2002).

[57] King D.E., Mainous A.G. 3rd, Carnemolla M., Everett C.J., Adherence to healthy lifestyle habits in US adults, 1988–2006. *Am. J. Med.* 122(6),528–534 (2009).

[58] Rimm E.B., Williams P., Fosher K., Criqui M., Stampfer M.J., Moderate alcohol intake and lower risk of coronary heart disease, meta-analysis of effects on lipids and haemostatic factor. *British Medical Journal.* 319 (7224), 1523–1528 (1999).

[59] Park H, Kim K. Association of alcohol consumption with lipid profile in hypertensive men. *Alcohol and Alcoholism.* 47(3), 282-287 (2012).

[60] Fuchs C.S., Stampfer M.J., Colditz G.A. et al., Alcohol consumption and mortality among women. *N Engl J Med.* 332(19), 1245 - 1250 (1995).

[61] Haynes S.G., Czajkowski S.M., Psychosocial and environmental correlates of heart disease. In: *Cardiovascular Health and Disease in Women*, Douglas PS (Ed), Saunders, Philadelphia p.269 (1993).

[62] Wassertheil-Smoller S., Shumaker S., Ockene J., et al. Depression and cardiovascular sequelae in postmenopausal women. The Women's Health Initiative (WHI). *Arch Intern Med.* 164 (3), 289-298 (2004).

[63] Mallik S., Spertus J.A., Reid K.J. et al., Depressive symptoms after acute myocardial infarction: evidence for highest rates in younger women. *Arch Intern Med.* 166 (8), 876–883 (2006).

[64] Egede L.E., Major depression in individuals with chronic medical disorders: prevalence, correlates and association with health resource utilization, lost productivity and functional disability. *Gen Hosp Psychiatry.* 29 (5), 409–416 (2007).

[65] Carney R.M., Freedland K.E., Miller G.E., Jaffe A.S., Depression as a risk factor for cardiac mortality and morbidity: a review of potential mechanisms. *J Psychosom Res.* 53 (4), 897–902 (2002).

[66] Everson-Rose S.A., Lewis T.T., Psychosocial factors and cardiovascular diseases. *Annu Rev Public Health.* 26, 469–500 (2005).

[67] Gehi A., Haas D., Pipkin S., Whooley M.A.n Depression and medication adherence in outpatients with coronary heart disease: Findings from the Heart and Soul Study. *Arch Intern Med.* 165 (21), 2508–2513 (2005).

[68] Hansson G.K., Inflammation, atherosclerosis, and coronary artery disease. *N. Engl. J. Med.* 352(16), 1685–1695 (2005).

[69] Maradit-Kremers H., Crowson C.S., Nicola P.J. et al., Increased unrecognized coronary heart disease and sudden deaths in rheumatoid arthritis: a population-based cohort study. *Arthritis Rheum.* 52(2), 402–411 (2005).

[70] Man S.F., van Eeden S., Sin D.D., Vascular risk in chronic obstructive pulmonary disease: role of inflammation and other mediators. *Can. J. Cardiol.* 28(6), 653–661 (2012).
[71] Emerging Risk Factors Collaboration, Kaptoge S, Di Angelantonio E, et al. C-reactive protein concentration and risk of coronary heart disease, stroke, and mortality: an individual participant meta-analysis. *Lancet.* 375 (9709), 132- 140 (2010).
[72] Rifai N., Buring J.E., Lee I.M., Manson J.E., Ridker P.M., Is C-reactive protein specific for vascular disease in women? *Ann. Intern. Med.* 136 (7), 529–533 (2002).
[73] Weiner D.E., Tighiouart H., Amin M.G. et al., Chronic kidney disease as a risk factor for cardiovascular disease and all-cause mortality: a pooled analysis of community-based studies. *J Am Soc Nephrol.* 15 (5), 1307–1315 (2004).
[74] Yu M.K., Katon W., Young B.A., Associations between sex and incident chronic kidney disease in a prospective diabetic cohort. *Nephrology* (Carlton). 20(7), 451-458 (2015).
[75] Stec J.J., Silbershatz H., Tofler G.H. et al., Association of fibrinogen with cardiovascular risk factors and cardiovascular disease in the Framingham Offspring Population. *Circulation.* 102 (14), 1634-1648.
[76] Karalliedde J., Viberti G., Microalbuminuria and cardiovascular risk. *Am J of Hypertens.* 17(10), 986-993 (2004).
[77] Zylberstein D.E., Bengtsson C., Björkelund C. et al., Serum homocysteine in relation to mortality and morbidity from coronary heart disease: a 24-year follow-up of the population study of women in Gothenburg. *Circulation.* 109 (5), 601- 606 (2004).
[78] Hu F.B., Grodstein F., Hennekens C.H. et al., Age at natural menopause and risk of cardiovascular disease. *Arch Intern Med.* 159 (10), 1061-1066 (1999).
[79] Colditz G.A., Willett W.C., Stampfer M.J. et al., Menopause and the risk of coronary heart disease in women. *N Engl J Med.* 316(18), 1105- 1110 (1987).
[80] Mack W.J., Slater C.C., Xiang M. et al. Elevated subclinical atherosclerosis associated with oophorectomy is related to time since

menopause rather than type of menopause. *Fertil Steril.* 82, 391-397 (2004).

[81] Howard B.V., Kuller L., Langer R. et al., Risk of cardiovascular disease by hysterectomy status, with and without oophorectomy: the Women's Health Initiative Observational Study. *Circulation.* 111(12), 1462 – 1470 (2005).

[82] Rossouw J.E., Anderson G.L., Prentice R.L. et al., Risks and benefits of estrogen plus progestin in healthy postmenopausal women: principal results From the Women's Health Initiative randomized controlled trial. *JAMA*. 288 (3), 321-333 (2002).

[83] Hulley S, Grady D, Bush T et al. Randomized trial of estrogen plus progestin for secondary prevention of coronary heart disease in postmenopausal women. Heart and Estrogen/progestin Replacement Study (HERS) Research Group. *JAMA*. 280(7), 605- 613 (1998).

[84] Grady D., Herrington D., Bittner V. et al., Cardiovascular disease outcomes during 6.8 years of hormone therapy: Heart and Estrogen/progestin Replacement Study follow-up (HERS II). *JAMA.* 288(1), 49- 57 (2002).

[85] Canoy D., Beral V., Balkwill A. et al., Age at menarche and risks of coronary heart and other vascular diseases in a large UK cohort. *Circulation.* 131(3), 237-244 (2015).

[86] Charalampopoulos D., McLoughlin A., Elks C.E., Ong K.K., Age at menarche and risks of all-cause and cardiovascular death: a systematic review and meta-analysis. *Am J Epidemiol*. 180(1), 29-40 (2014).

[87] Lakshman R., Forouhi N.G., Sharp S.J. et al., Early age at menarche associated with cardiovascular disease and mortality. *J Clin Endocrinol Metab.* 94 (12), 4953 – 4960 (2009).

[88] Lidegaard Ø., Løkkegaard E., Jensen A. et al., Thrombotic stroke and myocardial infarction with hormonal contraception. *N Engl J Med.* 366(24), 2257- 2266 (2012).

[89] Croft P., Hannaford P.C., Risk factors for acute myocardial infarction in women: evidence from the Royal College of General Practitioners' oral contraception study. *BMJ.* 298, 165 – 168 (1989).

[90] Rosenberg L., Palmer J.R., Rao R.S., Shapiro S., Low-dose oral contraceptive use and the risk of myocardial infarction. *Arch Intern Med.* 161(8), 1065-1070 (2001).

[91] Ahmed R., Dunford J., Mehran R. et al., Pre-eclampsia and future cardiovascular risk among women: a review. *J Am Coll Cardiol.* 63 (18), 1815 – 1822 (2014).

[92] Harreiter J., Dovjak G., Kautzky-Willer A., Gestational diabetes and cardiovascular risk after pregnancy. *Womens Health.* 10(1), 91-108 (2014).

[93] Oliver-Williams C.T., Heydon E.E., Smith G.C., Wood A.M., Miscarriage and future maternal cardiovascular disease: a systematic review and meta-analysis. *Heart.* 99 (22), 1636-1644 (2013).

[94] Robbins C.L., Hutchings Y., Dietz P.M. et al., History of preterm birth and subsequent cardiovascular disease: a systematic review. *Am J Obstet Gynecol.* 210 (4), 285-297 (2014).

[95] Wilson P.W., D'Agostino R.B., Levy D., Belanger A.M., Silbershatz H, Kannel WB. Prediction of coronary heart disease using risk factor categories. *Circulation.* 97(18), 1837–1847 (1998).

[96] D'Agostino R.B. Sr, Grundy S., Sullivan L.M., Wilson P., CHD Risk Prediction Group. Validation of the Framingham coronary heart disease prediction scores: results of a multiple ethnic groups investigation. *JAMA.* 286(2), 180–187 (2001).

[97] Ridker P.M., Buring J.E., Rifai N., Cook N.R., Development and validation of improved algorithms for the assessment of global cardiovascular risk in women: the Reynolds Risk Score. *JAMA.* 297(6), 611–619 (2007).

[98] Goff D.C. Jr, Lloyd-Jones D.M., Bennett G. et al., 2013 ACC/AHA guideline on the assessment of cardiovascular risk: a report of the American College of Cardiology/American Heart Association Task Force on Practice Guidelines. *Circulation.* 129(25 Suppl 2), S49-S73 (2014).

[99] Hsia J., Rodabough R.J., Manson J.E., et al., Evaluation of the American Heart Association cardiovascular disease prevention guideline for women. *Circ Cardiovasc Qual Outcomes*. 3, 128 -134 (2010).

INDEX

C

H

I

L

M

N

O

P

Q

R

S

T

U

V

W

Y